THE MAN IN THE MIRROR & OTHER STRANGERS

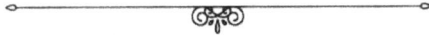

Looking at Alzheimer's Disease through the Life and Experiences of a Caregiver

Jenny Zimmer

The Man In The Mirror

Who is he?
Who was that man in my bathroom
The one who was looking at me this morning?
I don't like him – I don't want him here.
He wants to hurt me; he will hurt you too.
He's always looking at me… Get him out!

I turned you away from the mirror
Away from the image that stared back at you
The scary one – the stranger.
The man you don't like.
I soothed you – told you it would be OK
That I'd make him leave.
He couldn't hurt us then.

You quieted down
Then you went out onto the porch where you sat,
Smiling as you watched birds at the feeder
And you drank your third cup of coffee.
I went quietly into the house
And draped a towel over the mirror in your bathroom
Then… just to be safe,
I also covered the mirror by our front door
And the big one in the bedroom as well.

Now he's gone and he won't come back
You needn't fear the strange man
Who was in the bathroom this morning,
Looking at you, threatening you,
That dangerous man in the mirror
Who was watching you today.

©Jenny Zimmer 2022

Praise for 'The Man in the Mirror'

"The Man In The Mirror and Other Strangers is a very personal accounting of a caregiver's journey in dealing with a loved one with Alzheimer's. The author gives lots of self-help suggestions for anyone who is providing caregiving. Captivating read!"

-Sharon Perrino (Retired School Administrator/Caregiver)

"Jenny Zimmer is a master at reaching deep into a heart and writing so that the reader feels the emotions she hopes they will find helpful and reassuring. This book evolved to encourage other caretakers of loved ones with Alzheimer's on their journey. Her insights and demonstrated care should do that with an emphasis on "love". I enjoyed every page!"

-Barbara Kallmeyer (Jenny's writing friend)

"Jenny, I had the opportunity to read your book this afternoon. I think you did an incredible job of conveying the physical and emotional hardships of being a caregiver. However, I think the book is much more than a guide for care givers, I think it is a life guide for all of us. As I read your book, I was reminded that we never know what life has in store so we should cherish the moments we have together. I found your book to be a lesson in loving, caring, and focusing on the things within our control. Your book was emotionally moving and truly inspiring. You did a wonderful job."

-John Tepe (Executive Director at the care facility where Jenny's husband was for 16 months)

"Jenny has written an inspiring story about a devastating disease and its effects on the caregiver. The manuscript held my attention from the first word to the last. I believe this book will help other caregivers who seek to find someone who understands the difficulties ahead and suggests ways to face many of the problems. "The Man in The Mirror" is actually a love story, authentic and touching, but realistic as well. Bravo!"

-Noel Zeiser (Facilitator of Green Township Writers Group and Author of "The Pearl Street Flood" & "Salute the Moon")

"I found this book to be beautifully crafted, brutally honest, touchingly poignant, and filled with wisdom and grace. It speaks not only about the difficulties of Alzheimer's but also about the character and love of the author. Sharing your personal story will inspire others to approach the trials of loss and grief with courage and hope. Beautifully done."

"This book is so beautifully written. It brought tears to my eyes. Thank you for having the courage to share your journey in such as honest, yet loving way! Your unwavering love for your husband shines throughout the book. He was lucky to have you in both the good and not so good years. I know everyone will benefit from reading this book."

Table of Contents

Praise for 'The Man in the Mirror' ....

Dedication i

Foreword – An Alzheimer's Reading List.........................ii

Introduction iii

Victim, Not Patient 6

Senility or Alzheimer's – What's the Difference?.................8

Alzheimer's vs. Other Types of Dementia 12

The 'Yardman' 17

The Sharp Turn Downward 22

The Evolution – A Wife to a Caregiver 27

Dealing with the Storm 31

Our Treasures 36

Caregiver Rule 1..42

The Bond Between the Victim and the Caregiver 48

My Husband's Keeper...51

Finding a New Normal 54

Broken Pieces of a Favorite Vase 57

Going Through the Holidays 60

5 Caregiver Rules 63

Tinker, Tailor, Soldier, Spy… 68

A Life that's Mourned 72

Attrition 76

My Shrinking World..78

Questions that No Book can Answer 83

Strangers in Our House? 85

A Drastic Change Imminent 89

I Have to Let You Go… 92

A Cold Wind Blows 94

You've Got A Friend In Me 96

The Two of Us 99

The Things We Do for Love 103

Was He Okay Out There? 106

Why Him? 110

Limitations and Fears 112

The Big Band 40's 114

Savor the Good Moments 116

My Last Moments With Him 119

The Aftermath 125

I Miss You… 129

Ode of the Broken Heart 131

I Smile Because It Happened 134

Pictures of Al and Me 139

About the Author 143

Dedication

This book is dedicated to all the tired, stressed, and often overwhelmed caregivers who work so tirelessly to make life better for someone who can no longer take care of themselves.

God bless you all and give you strength!

Foreword – An Alzheimer's Reading List

- "The 36-Hour Day" by Nancy L. Mace, MA and Peter V. Rabins, MD, MPH
- "Is It Alzheimer's" by Peter Rabins, MD, MPH
- "Learning to Speak Alzheimer's" by Joanne Koenig-Coste and Robert N. Butler, MD
- "The Caregiver's Guide to Dementia: Practical Advice for Caring for Yourself and Your Loved One" by Gail Weatherill, RN
- "Loving Someone Who Has Dementia" by Pauline Boss
- "The Alzheimer's Answer Book: Professional Answers to More Than 250 Questions about Alzheimer's and Dementia" by Charles Atkins
- "A Caregiver's Guide to Dementia" by Janet Yagoda Shagam

Introduction

If anyone had told me a few years ago that I would one day author a book about Alzheimer's disease, I'd have thought it was a bad attempt at humor. Yet here I am today, writing about Alzheimer's; the disease, and the related events that completely turned my life around.

I'll begin by saying that numerous books, papers, and articles have been written about this disease. Doctors and other medical professionals have generally penned this literature with a lot of supporting research on the disease. Some have been authored by those involved in caring for someone with Alzheimer's.

Many professionals are working to discover what causes the disease and diligently seeking a way to prevent it, arrest it, and hopefully, someday find a way to cure it. Unfortunately, there are no answers to their questions at this time, even though a substantial amount of time, money, and research hours have been dedicated to the project.

I am not a clinician and therefore cannot offer opinions on what causes Alzheimer's, nor could I suggest possible treatments or cures. However, I have learned some important things about the disease in the last several years. The things I've learned will, hopefully, help you as you find yourself going down the path of change that this dreadful disease created in your life.

If you are just beginning your journey as a caregiver to someone with Alzheimer's, I strongly recommend that you read some of these professional books and learn as much as you can about the disease. However, as a caregiver, it is also essential that you read this book (and others like it) to learn more about how this journey will affect you.

My husband had Alzheimer's, and I am writing this book to describe the journey we took; a journey that led me into the role of the caregiver as his disease progressed.

However, you may be caring for someone suffering from another disease or illness. If so, this book will also have some helpful information and encouraging words for you as you enter into the caregiver world. And, as noted above, I recommend reading articles, books, and searching the internet for information on the particular disease with which you are dealing. It will help you in understanding the disease your loved one is facing.

As I mentioned earlier, Alzheimer's affects different people in different ways, so obviously the ways in which I handled some of my fears and frustrations, and the myriad of problems that I encountered in caring for my husband, may not be helpful to you. Just keep in mind that you are strong and capable of dealing with the problems you will encounter; don't let the raw feelings that haunt you make you feel otherwise.

It is not my intent to depress or frighten you or in any way to make the journey you are beginning more difficult, or threatening. I just hope that by sharing my feelings of frustrations, hopelessness, and even anger, and by telling you about some of the ways I found to cope with my emotions, will offer you some support and encouragement to help you on your journey as a caregiver.

I hope that by talking about my experiences, I can somehow help others who find themselves in the heartbreaking situation of becoming a caregiver. I am also optimistic that learning of my struggles will help sustain someone who is presently going through their own journey, and will help them to remember that, as hard as it can get sometimes, the feelings, fears, sadness, and even anger that they experience are quite normal. These feelings should not be repressed; caregivers will need to deal with them in some manner to protect their own health.

Whether you are a new caregiver or someone already going down that path, this book will hopefully give you the strength and courage to deal with your complicated feelings, raw emotions, and hard days. I sincerely hope so.

1

Victim, Not Patient

Let me first say that Alzheimer's does not discriminate in choosing its victims!

I say victims because this terrible disease attacks and robs the individual – leaving confusion, fear, and emptiness in its wake. It robs its victims of the ability to do routine things like carrying on a conversation – because words generally will become elusive and foreign; it robs victims of the ability to comprehend numbers – therefore eliminating practices such as making a telephone call, calculating a tip, and telling time.

It steals a victim's dignity. Needing to have someone assist with, or perform, daily personal tasks such as showering, shaving (if you're a man), and even toileting. Help with brushing teeth or combing their hair may be necessary and can often be hard for the Alzheimer's victim to accept. Thankfully, having a family member, or a trusted and familiar caregiver, assist with these personal needs can decrease or even partially eliminate the embarrassment, discomfort, and/or irritation the Alzheimer's victim may feel.

A diagnosis of Alzheimer's changes relationships. It often forces wives, husbands, children, siblings, and others to become caregivers. It's of course a role most of us know nothing about and one with which we are generally unfamiliar. When placed in this role, we start to feel frustrated and helpless, not knowing what to do or how to help our loved one. We can no longer function in our familiar and comfortable roles as spouses, children, etc.

But over a period of time, many find themselves functioning in a caregiver's role. When the realization of that role change occurs, it is often difficult for the affected individual to accept. Not to mention, it gets even more difficult as the Alzheimer's disease progresses, and the caregiver role accelerates and expands.

The disease eventually robs and steals everything from its victim, and replaces those things with a vacuum where only the present moment exists. When that occurs, the victim will generally have few, if any, memories to recall and cherish. Victims become unable to perform simple tasks such as making a bed, throwing a ball, etc., because the thought process and memory associated with the task no longer exists.

2

Senility or Alzheimer's – What's the Difference?

The quick answer is that there is little or no difference; they are both identified as dementia.

In years past, memory loss was often chalked up to Senility or Old Age. People with symptoms of memory loss were generally treated with some measure of courtesy by physicians. Usually, they were not given medical advice or medication to address the symptoms. No one bothered to look for a root cause for the problem; they just identified aging as the reason.

Many people – both physicians and families of the patient – thought and accepted that memory problems were a part of the normal aging process. Doctors usually indicated to their patients that there was nothing they could have done to prevent their memory loss.

The senility diagnosis and the idea that it was an inevitable by-product of aging was usually accepted with little or no questions, and life went on much as before. However, the victim's family often tried to make some allowances in caring for grandma, grandpa, or another family member who had received this diagnosis.

Then, in later years, a French psychiatrist Philippe Pinel coined the term dementia, which literally means "out of one's mind". It was then commonly used in reference to mental health. The word dementia is a broad term for disorders that affect the brain.

By the end of the 19th century, the term "dementia" was restricted to people experiencing loss of cognitive ability. During this period, Dr. James Cowles Pritchard introduced the term "Senile Dementia" in his book, "Treatise on Insanity." Then, in 1906 Alzheimer's was identified as a major form of dementia.

There are several types of memory loss. It can be caused by conditions that include vascular and sleep problems, medications, etc. Alzheimer's is one form of memory loss; as of today, no one has yet pinpointed the cause of this particular type of memory loss.

In addition, several conditions can mimic symptoms of Alzheimer's disease, sometimes making it difficult to correctly diagnose. For example, bacterial infections can cause memory loss, confusion, and other cognitive problems that are similar to those of Alzheimer's.

Alzheimer's is reported to be the worst form of dementia. It is also the most prevalent form of memory loss today. The primary cause of Alzheimer's is widely believed to be just age, however, other causes may include:

- Lack of activity/exercise
- Family history
- Traumatic brain injury (note: Despite continuing testing/studies, professionals have not found any conclusive connection between head injuries and Alzheimer's. Studies in this area are ongoing)
- Lack of brain stimulation

Estimates dictate there are now 6.5 million people, age 65 or older, who suffer from Alzheimer's disease, and two-thirds of that number are women. The number of people suffering from Alzheimer's is rising dramatically. It is predicted that half a million people will be diagnosed with Alzheimer's in the year 2022 alone! In a paper authored by Dr. David Williams, M.D. in 2005, he stated that by 2050, one out of eight people will have Alzheimer's. Since that time predictions have changed and now indicate a higher percentage of people who are diagnosed with Alzheimer's.

I can't help but wonder if the incidents of Alzheimer's are actually rising so dramatically, or if maybe we are seeing the results of more awareness and better diagnostic tools. Regardless, it is a major health concern.

Although over the years, there have been significant breakthroughs, there is still testing in the form of medication and even in diagnostic procedures but as yet, we do not know what causes the disease and there are no preventive measures, as far as I've heard and known.

According to the Alzheimer's Association, studies are currently underway that are testing new ways to identify reliable biomarkers for Alzheimer's that will lead to future diagnoses, therapy, and prevention even before symptoms start. Other studies are looking at dietary factors that could lower the risk of Alzheimer's.

It's fair to say at this time, researchers are no closer to determining a cure for Alzheimer's than they were twenty years ago. Something in me is still hopeful though that there will, one day soon, be a breakthrough in not only treatment but also in prevention and a cure.

3

Alzheimer's vs. Other Types of Dementia

All dementia sufferers have memory loss to some degree and perhaps some loss of verbal expression as well as other manifestations of dementia, similar to victims of Alzheimer's. What differentiates Alzheimer's victims is the loss of ability to perform life functions such as dressing, eating, bathing, toileting, and basic hygiene without assistance.

Persons with Alzheimer's may also become non-verbal. This can occur at any point in the disease's progression. For example, a friend's husband, diagnosed with Alzheimer's in his mid-fifties, stopped talking within two years of diagnosis. My husband, officially diagnosed in October of 2016 at age eighty-three, was, if anything, more talkative at times. Early on in the disease, he was just as outgoing as he had been before his illness began. Of course, that all changed and he became less talkative as the disease progressed and affected his ability to communicate.

As with other diseases, Alzheimer's affects people in different ways and at different points in their decline. Experts say that Alzheimer's victims may live anywhere from two to twenty years after diagnosis, depending on their age when diagnosed. The number of years lived is also affected by how quickly the disease progresses, the victim's physical health, and their lifestyle.

A cousin of mine took care of her husband at home for eight years before placing him in a care facility where he died about two years later. He also became non-verbal. Like my friend's husband, he too was diagnosed at a younger age.

Another friend's wife was diagnosed with Alzheimer's in her mid-seventies, and she was able to function at a relatively high level for several years but declined rapidly in the year before her death from breast cancer.

As you can see from these few examples, this cruel disease is not only non-discriminatory in its choice of victims but also very unpredictable in terms of how it affects each person and the speed at which it progresses.

There's a lot of medical information out there for anyone interested in learning more about the disease. But, rather than some general do's, don'ts, and how-to's for the caregiver, there's not much information about how the disease affects the caregiver or, as I prefer to describe them, the *other* victim of the disease.

Only very general information is given in terms of what you, as a caregiver, can expect to experience in the way of feelings. While books and articles may offer some good general advice for first-time caregivers, I don't think anyone can prepare in advance for this role. You simply assume it, or in other words, you just grow into it gradually as the need confronts and surrounds you.

In this book, I'll share some of the ups, downs, highs, and lows that I have personally experienced as I morphed into the role of caregiver.

To begin, I'll just say, it isn't an easy transition. Caring for someone with Alzheimer's is incredibly stressful. Statistics indicate that more than 50% of caregivers die before the person they are caring for!

Although the primary, and often the first, noticeable symptom of Alzheimer's may be memory loss, this is just the beginning. Caregivers will, at some point, deal with other symptoms, which may include any or all of the following, depression, anxiety, paranoia, sleeplessness, aggression, hallucinations, poor judgment and bad behavior.

Some men will make inappropriate comments, use foul language, and may exhibit sexual aggression. Many men, and women too for that matter, will show a volatile temper and be threatening to others. Add to that the Alzheimer's victim's inability to perform many life functions such as dressing, eating, and using the bathroom.

There may be a time when your loved one won't know who you are, and that hurts. But, even if they don't know who you are, they somehow do know that you are someone they feel safe with and who is helping them. Fortunately, my husband knew me until the end of his life, and I feel certain he knew his sister.

Alzheimer's victims may easily become frightened, and the world around them can become quite threatening. For example, they do not like for someone to grab them or approach them from behind. They often are afraid of sitting down, feeling as if they might fall.

Many Alzheimer's patients are unsettled or disturbed by their image in the mirror. My cousin's husband was upset and frightened when seeing himself in the mirror. He thought it was another man in their house. He would curse and threaten to kill that man. His reaction caused a lot of anxiety for his wife and son. Eventually, they had to cover all mirrors and/or other reflective items in their house.

Many are afraid of water and will resist getting into the shower. When I talked to a professional about this, she told me that the patient may feel that when stepping into the shower, they are stepping/falling into a hole.

The last time I attempted to get my husband into the shower while he was still at home, he tried but just couldn't make himself step over the threshold. He told me that he felt 'the water was going to cut him to shreds'. I was later told that many Alzheimer's patients have this same fear about water.

4

The 'Yardman'

In late 2015 and early 2016, we began to suspect something more than normal forgetfulness was happening when my husband started having trouble communicating. He often couldn't find the words to express himself. He also had difficulty remembering names of people and objects. Often these were people that he had known for a long time or objects with which he was quite familiar. For a year, and possibly two prior to that time, he had started to experience memory issues, and they were getting noticeably worse.

As months passed, we observed other odd things, such as forgetting to put the car in park before turning off the engine, losing track of dates, etc. Then he began to have trouble telling time or even reading numbers, and he had a hard time staying focused on anything.

One day when he was writing checks, he asked me how to make an asterisk or "and" sign. I showed him and he practiced making it but couldn't do it very well. At that point, he was beginning to not trust himself to

17

write checks; he sometimes had difficulty signing his name. He asked me to start writing his checks, personal and business. Before much longer, I was managing all our personal and business activities.

He wasn't able to calculate the tip on restaurant checks. He had no concept of the value of money, often looking to me for help in knowing what denomination of money to use. Around that same time, he stopped answering the phone or making calls as he could not remember which buttons to push. He no longer knew how to turn the TV on or off and couldn't use the remote to change channels. I also noticed that he, someone who had always enjoyed the TV and especially western movies, exhibited less and less interest in any program.

Although an avid reader in the past, he now seldom picked up a book, newspaper, or magazine anymore. When he did, he had difficulty reading. He tried to continue reading but couldn't. Although he never indicated or admitted that he was having a problem and tried to keep up the pretense, it was quite noticeable. In time, he just stopped trying.

Alzheimer's victims are generally incredibly good at covering up their deficiencies, but that only lasts for a period of time, or until their deception is discovered.

I was extremely concerned and felt we should see a neurologist, but even suggesting that was difficult. I didn't want to upset him or in any way make him feel less than the man who was strong and capable, the man he'd always been.

At that time, I still didn't think of myself as a caregiver but rather as a helper... I was just helping my husband do the things he had done regularly but things that he now required some assistance in performing. Many of these things he now found difficult to do were simple and somewhat mindless tasks, such as filling the gas tank on the lawn tractor and mowing the grass.

We did find some ways to cope. For example, when he didn't remember how to start his Cub Cadet lawn tractor, I learned how to start and operate it by reading the operations manual. Then, hoping to help him remember how to do it, I photocopied pages of the manual that detailed how to start it. I highlighted the three important steps, laminated the pages, and hung them in a conspicuous place next to where the tractor was stored.

I don't believe he ever looked at those pages, but I did, and I soon found myself quite comfortable using the mower. That was a good thing because by late summer, he had not only forgotten how to operate the mower, but he had lost all interest in doing anything in the yard.

He would usually lie on the couch and sleep while I was in the yard. I didn't have to worry about leaving him in the house alone but nonetheless, I would go in to check on him a couple of times while working outside.

I found myself doing it all – in addition to the yard, I was also doing all the cooking, laundry, keeping the house clean, taking care of bills, grocery shopping, etc. I tried to keep things normal.

By this time, I was beginning to feel some pressure. I sometimes found myself running up against things that I didn't know how to do, and that was upsetting to me. I sometimes felt a little resentful that I had to cope with the things he had always just taken care of. I had to assume responsibility for the yard and landscaping, and I needed to learn some new things. Suddenly I realized that I had become the 'yardman' without even knowing it. I was starting to feel overwhelmed.

But I still didn't consider myself a caregiver. In fact, that thought didn't even occur to me.

Making the bed in the morning or turning it back in the evening, things we had always done together, became difficult for him; he couldn't remember the task sequence and would become agitated with me when I tried to show him. He would often accuse me of changing my mind about how things were done, and he would simply walk away, leaving me to complete the task alone.

Changes in him became more noticeable and seemed to occur more quickly. It seemed that more and more areas of our lives were affected.

I was also becoming increasingly worried about him. I couldn't help but wonder if his problems were caused by something we were doing but shouldn't be doing, or something we should be doing but weren't.

Were the vitamins and supplements that he took on a daily basis causing these problems? Were there new vitamins and/or supplements that could alleviate or lessen his memory problems? Was there something in our lifestyle that was causing the changes in him? What reason could there be? My bewilderment was intense.

And behind this worry was a constant fear in my mind... could he possibly have Alzheimer's?

My world began to shrink along with his, but in a vastly different way.

5

〰︎〰︎

The Sharp Turn Downward

We began to see other changes in him.

One day I mentioned the idea of seeing a specialist about the memory issues he was experiencing. I mentioned the name of a doctor who specialized in, and was well known and respected for her work with all forms of brain disorders.

We had already visited our Primary Care Physician three times with our concerns, and he had, at one point, ordered a brain MRI. When the test results came back, our doctor told us that the MRI showed only 'age-related changes'. When I questioned what that meant, he explained that it was 'a normal slowing down' due to aging. We weren't happy with this explanation but... where were we to turn to get information that might explain it better?

The specialist that I mentioned to my husband had been recommended by a friend who was a nurse and a golfing friend of mine. The recommendation came through a conversation one day. Another friend, whose mother was going through the same type of memory problems as my husband, had asked who would be the best doctor for her mother to see for her memory issues.

I knew that my husband needed to see a doctor and, although we hadn't discussed it, he had mentioned several times that he wished he could 'get his words back'. I was now hopeful that he would agree to see the specialist my friend had recommended. I felt that passing the information about the doctor on to my husband would be easier now since I could do it under the guise of repeating the conversation between our nurse friend and the friend who was seeking help for her mother.

When I told him about this doctor, he showed some interest and said he would like to talk to my friend about it. I called her that evening and asked if she could stop by after work sometime in the next few days.

Two days later, we sat down with her and learned more about the doctor she had endorsed. She told us a little about what we could expect when we saw the doctor. I called the next day for an appointment and got one scheduled but, it was for a date three months away.

When our appointment date arrived, we had to complete several questionnaires and an assessment of his overall condition before we saw the doctor. Technicians in the office did a lot of testing to begin with. I was sent in to visit with a social worker while my husband was being evaluated. The doctor spoke with both of us, and she also did several tests to determine his physical, mental, and emotional condition.

She explained that there could be several reasons for his memory loss, including medications. She reviewed the few medications he was taking and immediately took him off the one he had been taking for several years to control his anxieties. She said that it could cause, or add to, memory issues. She replaced it with a different medication that would not have that effect on him.

At the end of that two-hour appointment, the doctor recommended that he have a brain MRI which she would compare to the one our Primary Care Physician had ordered a year prior. She also wanted him to have a sleep study done to determine whether sleep apnea was causing, or contributing to, his memory loss. She ordered a complete blood workup and a spinal puncture. Her nurse set up appointments for these tests to be done that month, and another appointment with the doctor was scheduled shortly.

It was interesting to learn that Alzheimer's disease could be diagnosed through a spinal puncture. In contrast, previously it was only diagnosed through an autopsy or brain surgery. This method was new and, in 2016, there were only two labs in the United States that could analyze the spinal fluid and determine whether or not the patient had Alzheimer's. Diagnosing this disease was a huge breakthrough in the Alzheimer's research process.

At our appointment, based on the test results, my husband was officially diagnosed with Late-Onset Alzheimer's. When I asked what stage he was in, the doctor said she liked re-testing a patient in six months and then comparing the two tests before determining the stage.

The doctor prescribed 5 mg daily of a popular medication which, she explained, could possibly slow the progression of the disease and give him up to two additional years of quality life. He was scheduled for an appointment and follow-up evaluation in six months.

Based on what I had read and observed, I also mentioned to her that he seemed to be in the middle stage of the disease, and the doctor nodded yes. I then added that I thought he was more than halfway through that middle stage, and she again nodded yes. So, we now had some idea of where he was in his journey with the disease.

Unfortunately, a side effect of the medication she prescribed was a runny nose. When she upgraded to a 10 mg tablet, that side effect became so uncomfortable and distracting that he couldn't tolerate it. So when we saw the doctor six months later, she moved him back down to 5 mg, which decreased the severity of the side effect. But the runny nose finally became so distracting, and it irritated him so much that I took him off the medication altogether. I advised the doctor of my action and told her that I didn't feel it was helping him in any way. It was just an uncomfortable complication and one that he didn't need. She understood.

By this point in time, he had become less active. He was sleeping several hours each day while also sleeping through the night. I was concerned about the amount of sleep he was getting and asked the doctor about it. Her answer was that it was a symptom associated with Alzheimer's and common for someone who suffered from the disease.

I was also observing other changes in his behavior and became more concerned each day. I constantly worried about what was in his future. What could I do to protect him?

Our life had taken a sharp turn downward.

6

The Evolution – From Wife to Caregiver

This book is not meant to be just about my husband's illness as he sank further into the Alzheimer's abyss, but rather it is about how this disease affected his life and how it affected me – his wife, companion, and later on, his caregiver. But before I share my feelings in this path of evolving into the caregiver role for my husband, it is necessary for me to relate much of his journey as well.

I wrote earlier about how Alzheimer's robs and steals from its victims; it doesn't stop there. It also victimizes the caregiver. More so when the caregiver is a family member who can't just walk away from all of it at the end of the day, someone who lives with it 24 hours a day, every day of the week for as long as the person they are caring for is alive.

At what point did I realize I was a caregiver? It took a while, several months in fact, to acknowledge that the changes brought into our lives by his illness were also changing me and my everyday life.

I guess the first clue was when I began to feel the agonizing realization that I was losing my freedom.

I was hesitant to go out, even for a brief period of time, without having someone stay with him. I wasn't, at that time, worried about his leaving the house or doing anything to harm himself. But I was concerned because of his lack of interest in doing anything such as reading, watching TV, or anything else that would help him pass the time. I thought the time he spent alone would seem so long and lonely for him since he had no concept of time. And I didn't want him to ever feel abandoned.

The only family close by was his sister. She would come over to stay with him when I had an appointment or when I went to my book club once a month. She would prepare his lunch, look at old photo albums with him, and they would walk around the yard. I hated to ask her to come too often since she had a life of her own – a home, and a husband to care for. Thank God she was willing and available to help then and even more later on when things became more difficult.

That was the time when I started to feel like a caregiver.

I wasn't even able to go out grocery shopping or to the post office without someone having to come over to stay with him. And even if I did leave him with someone, I wouldn't stop worrying about him. Eventually, all of this prevented me from going out altogether. It just seemed easier to put things off than to ask for help. So ultimately, anything that wasn't absolutely necessary was postponed, sometimes for several weeks or even indefinitely.

During the initial stages of my caregiver role, I once left him alone to run to the grocery store only to come back 30 minutes later to find him descending the stairs, wearing his coat and hat, heading for his car in the garage. When I entered through the door, he said, "I was worried about you and was going to look for you."

I was lucky to catch him before he left. We had averted what could have been a disaster had he left in his car. From this incident, I realized two particularly important things. First, he needed to have someone with him all the time, and second, I needed to hide his car keys so there wouldn't be any possibility of him leaving.

After that occurrence, my solution was to order groceries online in the evening and then pick them up early the next morning before he was awake. That worked out well and resolved the issue for me.

It was no longer safe for him to drive as his judgment had become impaired. Based on the doctor's recommendation, I now had to do all the driving. At first, I got a lot of criticism from him which made me nervous and sometimes left me feeling pretty aggravated. Sometimes I even felt resentment at being placed in this position.

Quite often I felt uncomfortable driving, especially when I wasn't certain about directions. I had always depended on him to know how to get wherever we were going. Oddly enough, he did remember some routes and could sometimes help me find my way when I was unsure. Eventually, we both got used to me doing all the driving.

7

Dealing with the Storm

It was hard for me to accept or to even acknowledge the feelings this life-altering turmoil generated in me. I was filled with feelings of anxiety, incompetence, frustration, hurt, anger and fear, and I really needed to vent. I needed to talk to someone, but who?

Although two of my closest friends, along with my son, daughter-in-law, and my sister-in-law were always willing to listen, I still struggled with my feelings and didn't feel comfortable talking about them. For some reason, I found it difficult to verbalize what our daily routine was like, and how the changes in his health had leached out into every aspect of our life.

His health deeply troubled me at times, and I couldn't help but be concerned over my ability to handle everything as well. In a desperate attempt to vent my feelings and better understand them, I started writing a blog shortly after that initial meeting with the doctor. It was not made public but was only available to be viewed by selected people. Somehow I found it easier to write about my feelings and concerns than to verbalize them.

My intention in writing the blog was solely to have a place where I could express my feelings as they were becoming difficult for me to deal with. I knew I needed some outlet, a proper kind of catharsis. In that blog (http://www.fohshallqueen@wordpress.com), I tried to describe my feelings and fears; I received a lot of supportive feedback from friends and family, many of whom had not known, up to that time, what was happening to us. Or, if they did know, they hadn't realized the extent of his illness or the changes that were occurring in our lives.

At first, I didn't share the information about the blog with his sister or others in his family because I harbored a fear that they would be unhappy that I was disclosing his illness.

For those of you who may just now be getting into a caregiver's role, I have shared some of those blog posts here so you can see how I dealt with the raw feelings that I was experiencing during that time.

This was my first blog post:

June 22, 2016

Handling Life's Changes

Change – constant and often unexpected! Our lives go along for years with changes that are mostly positive ones.... marriage, children, a new home, career advancements, etc. Happy changes!

Then, one day, the unexpected happens.... change that is not positive but change that brings something new and frightening into our lives. I'm talking about change that occurs with the advent of memory loss, confusion, etc. to a loved one. What to do? How do we address it with our loved one? Dare we say that we notice the changes and are concerned? Can we suggest doctor visits/tests?

Two years ago, things changed with my husband, most noticeable the ability to find words sometimes and dealing with anything that contained numbers. Writing checks became something he wasn't able to do, he couldn't remember how to make certain numbers, how to state an amount and even, at times, how to sign his name.

In the past two years more things have changed, and he is a vastly different man than the one I have known for years. He is still the man I love, and I want to help him in any way I can. But in my dealing with the changes occurring with him, I am also changing.

I have had to become the decision maker, the money manager, the one to remember when things need to be done, etc. In many ways, I feel like I'm living alone. It's scary, what if I don't make the right decision about something, don't take care of something that needs to be done, or a bill that needs to be paid.

I pray every day for my husband, and I also pray daily for me, for the strength and courage to deal with the changes coming into my life and I ask God to give me the wisdom I need to take care of things.

Writing and publishing that first blog post allowed me to release some part of the burden that was pressing down on me. I received some very encouraging feedback from those who had been invited to read it. I purposely did not use his name, or mine, in my blog posts since I didn't want anyone to identify us and, as I mentioned before, I wasn't sure how his family would feel about me sharing these very personal things.

It was only later in the year that I finally told his family about the blog. I even sent each of them a link to it. I was relieved that they all now knew about his illness and the extent of his decline. I was thankful for their prayers and the concern voiced in their very loving and supportive feedback.

8

Our Treasures

We continued to have good days when things seemed pretty normal, and then there were also the bad days where he was pretty agitated, testy, sometimes even quiet, and generally not showing much interest in anything.

On the good days, he did enjoy sitting outside, sometimes for several hours. I often took our lunch outside and we would sit in our gazebo, listening to the birds, talking, and admiring the flowers as we had a leisurely lunch.

I think the moment when I knew our lives had crossed into an irrevocable phase was the day when my husband and I were in the kitchen with the radio playing, and we danced...

On July 11, 2016, I posted the following to my blog:

One Day to The Next

I love the radio and turning it on is generally one of the first things I do each morning. That has been my practice for as long as I can remember. In these days of Satellite radio, I turn to Channel 69, a station that plays a variety of music, all of which is easy on the ears.

One morning this past winter it seemed the music was especially good and, as we cleaned up the dishes after breakfast, my husband took me in his arms and, with the sunshine streaming into the room, we slowly danced in our kitchen.

As we danced a deep sadness filled me, tears came to my eyes and I tightened my arms around him; I knew at that moment that it was the beginning of the end to the life we had known up to that time. The music ended and we stood for a moment, not speaking, holding each other tightly. I think we both knew.

We have lots of "good days" or days when things seem to be pretty normal if we don't delve too deeply into the little things that occur. I treasure every one of those days and know that I am lucky to get them.

There isn't a day when I don't somehow question my ability to deal with the changes occurring in my life; there are no days that I don't pray for guidance, and no days when I'm not thankful for the dances that we've had up till now.

That kitchen dance was both an ending and a beginning for us. It was our moment of truth.

The cousin that I mentioned earlier told me that her moment of truth was when she accidentally overturned a bucket of water as she scrubbed the floor and spilled the water. As she began to clean it up, her husband, whose Alzheimer's disease was pretty far along at the time, had observed the spill. He wrapped his arms around her and said, "Don't worry, it'll be alright." She began to cry and said to him, "No, nothing will ever be alright again."

And my friend who cared for her husband in their home for thirteen years told me that they did not realize the full extent of his occasional memory lapses because, after all, he was only in his mid-fifties and healthy. But then a defining moment came when he was fired from his job for making a mistake that cost the company quite a bit. She learned then that he had made earlier mistakes that had been swished away as accidents. Although my friend's husband was never formally diagnosed with Alzheimer's, they knew he was a victim of the disease.

I believe that there is a defining moment in the lives of all Alzheimer's victims as well as for those close to them. My definition of a defining moment is the time when realization hits and when they, the victim, and their loved ones, begin their new, sometimes terrifying journey into the world of Alzheimer's.

My life had become quite stressful. I was often at my wit's end and felt quite lost and lonely; I struggled, not knowing what I could do to help him.

But, even in times like this, some very humorous things can occur. These things can provide comic relief and can lighten moods. But as the disease progresses, chances are that those humorous incidents will lessen or even disappear, leaving us with the memories of such episodes.

This one time for example, we were just returning from a trip to the post office, I pulled into our driveway and unfastened his seatbelt so he could get out, but the entire time he just sat there smiling. When I told him to get out, he simply replied, "Okay," but he didn't budge. He wouldn't get out of the car despite my coaxing and pleading. I finally got out, walked around the car to the passenger side, and tried to get him out myself; I even tried to lift his feet and physically help him out of the car, but that didn't work either.

There was a gleaming smile on his face the whole time, seemingly enjoying it all. After several more minutes of pleading with him, he decided to get out. As I left him standing there, I walked around to get in on the driver's side but when I sat down, there he was... sitting in the passenger seat again!

Feeling totally frustrated by that time, I got out of the car and went back around to the passenger side, only to beg him to get out. But, once again, he didn't move. After a full five minutes of this, I had enough and I ended up raising my voice, "GET OUT OF THE CAR!" Surprisingly, he did. I climbed back into the driver's seat and pulled the car into the garage as he waited there in the driveway. Then he casually walked into the house with me as if nothing unusual had happened. Neither of us brought it up when we walked inside or even later that day.

While I was making our dinner that evening, I realized how funny this incident had actually been. I had a good chuckle out of it and even shared it with my friends in an e-mail. They also found it funny.

Then, later that evening when I was getting him settled for the night, he looked up at me with a sweet smile, patted me on the cheek and said, "I like you so much better than that other girl." I knew he was referring to "that other girl", the one who had raised her voice at him earlier. That also gave me a good chuckle. I kissed his cheek and said, "Goodnight."

Several months later when he was in a care facility, I shared that story with the other participants in the Support Group and, to my surprise, they all laughed at it as well. The facilitator even told me that she has repeated this story over and over at various places and that everyone enjoys it and that it generally brings back memories of humorous moments in their lives as caregivers.

There were other moments in my life, filled with funny questions, observations, or comments that made me and my husband both laugh. But with those, there were also many occurrences that were poignant, sad, frustrating, and disheartening for us. We felt them all and dealt with each of them as they surfaced. But the most important part about this journey was that we clung to each other, and even though we knew that this journey would not take us to a happy conclusion, we were content with what we had.

Here's another bit of humor... My cousin told me that, one time while she was caring for her husband at home, she wasn't feeling well and just wasn't up to cooking anything for him, so she made him a peanut butter and jelly sandwich that he ate without any protest.

This went on for three days, PB&J sandwiches for lunch, still no comment from him. Then later on, shortly after she had placed him in an assisted living facility, she said to him one day that the food there seemed pretty good. He looked at her and said, "Well, it beats peanut butter and jelly sandwiches." It still makes me chuckle.

9

◞◞◜◜

Caregiver Rule 1

My blog post from July 30, 2016, reads:

Definition of Change – To Make different – To Alter in Some Way

The changes in my husband's health have altered not only his life and lifestyle but mine and that of other close family members as well. I feel certain that our feelings of anger at the things happening to him and the sadness that we feel at losing parts of him, can't compare to the feelings of frustration and despair that he must feel.

Can you imagine not knowing the time or not knowing how long an hour is? Can you imagine getting up at 3 or 4 AM to shower and dress for a 10 AM appointment because you don't know what time it is? Those are some of the things he is dealing with. I've asked him to just trust me about the time to get up, to leave for appointments, etc. and he says that I have a weird clock.

I need to be able to comfort and re-assure him when he's feeling frustrated or upset; I need to watch my voice tone so that I don't sound bossy, critical, mean, or harsh; I need to remember that I am his life-preserver in what is now a stormy sea. I pray for wisdom and guidance as we go through each day.

After this episode, I crafted some ground rules for myself. One rule or, as I like to call it, my Caregiver's Rule #1 is to 'Always watch my tone of voice, keeping it friendly so that I don't appear to be bossy, critical, mean or harsh'. This was a good reminder for me.

But in this journey, I felt like I was losing myself as well. My feelings became more intense and complicated. It was normal for me to feel hurt, angry, annoyed, helpless, and lonely on any given day. I was sad most of the time. I was scared. The things that had previously held my interests or satisfied me proved futile in distracting me, even painting and writing. My life now revolved around him and his needs.

I think having these feelings come with the territory – dealing with unexpected changes around you can cause a variety of strong feelings to surface. How we choose to deal with these feelings offers a path to conquer them.

Then, on September 14, 2016, I posted this:

Where are the Tears?

There are plenty of reasons for tears in my life today, sadness, and yes, even anger at the changes that are affecting someone I love; frustration with my inability to help him; fear that I can't do this, that I'm not strong enough, or wise enough to manage the responsibility placed on me as a caregiver.

And even though I can see the changes in him and, in our daily life, I feel that there is still a level of denial that exists for me along with the hope that something, anything, will help him and make it all better. Yet, even with the sadness, anger, frustration, and fears, there haven't been any tears yet.

I can see that I am changing too. I am not the same person I was before, not the same person that found joy in so many things and who laughed a lot. Oh, I still find joy in life and I laugh but I am quieter, more thoughtful, and more serious. I am conscious of this happening to me and try to guard against it. I don't want to lose me. the person that I am!

So, where are the tears? I guess it's just not time for them yet but I can feel them getting closer and closer. So, one day soon I'm going to find a moment of solitude and let the sadness, anger, frustration, and fear pour out.

Thank God for family and for the friends who listen and encourage, who give me strength, and love. I know that regardless of the changes in my husband, in me, and in our life, they are there for us.

Maybe you'll break sooner than I did and cry your eyes out, hoping for all of this to be just a bad dream, or maybe you will find a path to handle the overwhelming feelings of sadness, loss, and helplessness that you have had for a while now. You need to look for ways to find that release sooner than later.

Check with the *Alzheimer's Association* for names of places where you can get some help. Your local chapter will also offer counseling and other programs that will help you cope with these overwhelming changes in your life.

Many churches and hospitals offer programs that provide you with the best information about agencies or services available in your area. My doctor recommended a couple of places to me and then had his assistant contact these places to set up appointments.

Some local agencies such as *Council on Aging* may provide services at little to no cost. If you are not successful at finding an agency to work with, or if finances are a problem, you may want to arrange for a family member or a friend to come to your house twice or more times a week to take care of your loved one, giving you some free time.

Whatever course you end up taking to get some help and some release, you must be certain that it doesn't affect your loved one negatively. If someone comes in to take care of your loved one, will they treat them kindly and be respectful of their limitations? Will they speak in a gentle manner and not scold, argue or yell under any circumstances? I believe that it is critical for the caregiver to have a patient and calm manner.

Things were not looking up, and we were seeing changes occur at, what seemed to me, a pretty fast pace. This post was written before we saw the doctor again.

I was anxious to see her and find out what we were dealing with. At the time, he was still able to communicate pretty well, except for times when he had difficulty in finding the correct words. But I could tell that he was getting more and more concerned and, on several occasions, he expressed, "I wish I could get my words back."

And all the time I was watching his health deteriorate, there wasn't a moment when I didn't feel helpless. I felt a deep and all-consuming sadness.

Here is an excerpt from my October 14, 2016, posting:

One Day at A Time

There are good days and others not so good....

... The past few weeks have had some moments when I wasn't sure I could manage what was coming. There have been days when things have not gone well and that caused a strain on our relationship. Hearing some of the things he says when he is upset or angry is hurtful and hard for me to accept but I'm learning not to retort or argue a point. After a while, things smooth out and he is once again the sweet, affectionate, and appreciative husband that I have lived with for the past thirty-seven years ...

10

~~~

The Bond Between the Victim and the Caregiver

As the disease progresses, it turns the victim's partner from a lover into a nice, yet a non-personal caregiver. It turns a relationship with previously tender moments and a loving behavior into what becomes a dependency – based on need and, to some degree, on trust. It's a working relationship with a bond between the Alzheimer's victim and the caregiver.

Even now I remember well the moment when I knew that Alzheimer's was not like other diseases. There were no preventative measures and no cure at all; there were only a couple of known medications that could possibly slow the progression of it. It affected both men and women, educated and uneducated, all ages, all levels of society, and all races. As I said before, the disease is not discriminating in its choice of victims.

As I mentioned earlier, Alzheimer's is the worst form of dementia. Although there is a lot of speculation about causes, treatments, and cures, as of today there is still no concrete evidence to support researchers in their quest to find answers.

In the meantime, the number of people with Alzheimer's continues to rise up drastically. Among the top ten causes of death in America, including cancer and heart disease, Alzheimer's is the only disease that cannot be prevented, cured, or even slowed down.

Our life as we knew it had ended the moment my husband became a victim. Our normal (pre-Alzheimer's) life was filled with tender moments. He and I used to work together in the house and the yard. For fun we would oftentimes just indulge in playing golf, going out with friends for dinner, attending plays, ball games and, when we wanted to just relax, we would have lunches together, sometimes just a beer in our gazebo as we enjoyed the flowers blooming in our garden and in the patio pots. We listened to the chirping of birds that came to our feeders and the bird baths. Looking back, that all seems so distant.

We used to have wonderful conversations on almost any topic you could name. He was an expert in European history, and I loved hearing him talk about events and/or rulers over the past years. He was also well-versed in alternative medicines, supplements, and herbal remedies.

We had so much love and affection and laughter in our marriage; our life was pleasant and good.

Seeing my husband slowly change from the happy, loving, and caring man that he once was into this sad and somewhat lifeless being that the disease left him to be was difficult to watch, and as harsh as it sounds, I would have preferred losing him to death rather than seeing this agonizingly slow deterioration. It hurt me to watch as my husband slowly lost everything that made him him, and having a front-row seat to the turmoil only made it worse.

A word of advice; treasure the moments that make you feel that things are back to the old, normal and sometime boring life you once had. Treasure those little moments filled with laughter, those tender moments, pleasant conversations, and meals. Each of these days is a gift from God!

11

My Husband's Keeper

Alzheimer's, like any debilitating disease, will generally bring new challenges and/or problems almost daily. And when they do arise, it is most often left for the caregiver to find a way to cope with the issue.

As an example, my husband, who was then about halfway through the middle stage of the disease, began not wanting to get into the shower. After several days, I had to practically force him to get in. While watching him closely after he got in, it occurred to me what was causing his behavior. It was simple really… he no longer knew how to turn the water on, or how to adjust the water temperature.

After thinking about how I might resolve the problem, it made sense to me to have him get into the shower before the water was turned on. Then, I could reach in, turn the water on, and adjust the temperature for him.

Of course, it was pretty obvious that I was helping him, and I felt uncomfortable doing it. I also felt like I needed to explain why I was doing it, which was something I didn't feel I could do. I didn't want him to know that I had noticed he was having a problem. So, I simplified it by getting into the shower first and then, when I stepped out, leaving the water on for him. That seemed to work better for a while.

However, getting him to step into the shower became increasingly difficult, regardless of my efforts. I then started getting into the shower with him, but he would stand back away from the water and only stood under it when I coaxed him. Even then, he would move away quickly, hardly giving me time to rinse the soap off of him.

One day, he really tried to step into the shower without my coaxing, but he would back away each time he tried. When I encouraged him to get in, he looked up at the water coming out of the shower head, then looked back at me and said, "I'm afraid it's going to just cut me to shreds." I held his robe for him, and we turned away; there would be no shower that day.

That just broke my heart! My 6-foot, 225 pound, hard-working, strong, athletic husband was feeling a fear so intense that he couldn't overcome it. I had to turn away so that he wouldn't see my despair.

Now I knew it was fear causing his hesitancy, and, not wanting to subject him to that fear any more often than necessary, I suggested that I give him a sponge bath. We tried it, but it didn't work well as he would become agitated sitting in the chair while I washed him.

That was when I crafted my Caregiver's Rule #2, which is to 'Accept the challenge or problem that has presented itself and then to look for, and find, a workable solution'. At this point, I still didn't fully recognize that I was functioning in a caregiver's role. We still had many good days, hours when we enjoyed a good laugh, and a tall drink while sitting in our gazebo, just talking and enjoying being together. We even had some conversations that weren't too far from what might be considered normal. We made plans for the future, and that was difficult for me because I knew in my heart that the things we planned would not be in the future that surely would be ours.

But for now, my goal was to help him get along in life, to make things easier for him, and to hopefully give him some joy. I wanted him to feel that he was still the man of the house, my protector, my security.

I also wanted and needed to take care of him.

12

Finding a New Normal

From my post on February 3, 2017:

Finding a New Normal

Our lives have taken a new direction recently. Where 10:30 or 11:00 PM bedtimes were the norm for us through the years, my husband now goes to bed at 9:00 PM and actually starts looking at the clock around 8:00 PM. Since I'm not ready for bed that early, I spend a couple of hours catching up on a project, reading, writing, etc.

Sleep habits have changed for both of us. Actually, my sleep pattern has changed dramatically with waking frequently after midnight or lights out, sometimes two, three or more times a night and then sleeping late the next morning. The new norm in our house is getting up at 9:00 AM, having a late breakfast and then a late lunch. I sometimes feel like I'm just treading water…. getting nowhere.

I ask God daily to help me know when, how, and how much help to give to my husband. I often have to hold back, letting him do things on his own. But it is

54

becoming more apparent that he needs my help with more things such as dressing and keeping track of his glasses. During the past two weeks I have noticed a decline in his abilities. We see the doctor in one more week and he will be re-tested so she will be able to give us her opinion as to the stage of his disease.

He is constantly tired and sleeps a lot. He naps after breakfast and in the afternoon then goes to bed early. I miss having conversations with him and I miss his company. I do try to involve him in decisions, but it is becoming increasingly difficult for him to understand what I'm asking of him.

So, yes, we have a new normal to our daily routine. I know that I am changing too as our lifestyle changes. I ask God for guidance, for peace, and calm to take me through each day and I try to pass that peace and calm along to my husband thereby making his day comfortable and happy.

Losing him is sad and my sadness is almost overwhelming at times.

I know that it's so hard for him especially when he knows that something is wrong and that it is getting worse. Oddly, his disease has brought us closer together. We share a love and closeness that is special and one which keeps us going day after day. My heart aches for him!

This poem expresses my feelings:

Discovery

Last night I stretched up my hands
And touched the stars above.
The moon smiled back when I looked at him
And the whole world shone with love.
But tonight, the stars have turned their faces,
And dark clouds hide the moon;
How did they all find out so fast
That sadness fills my heart's empty room.

©Jenny Zimmer 2007

13

Broken Pieces of a Favorite Vase

Each day was hard. <u>My freedom and my 'ME' time was non-existent; my life had changed so dramatically that I hardly knew who I was anymore.</u>

That sounds dramatic and hopeless, but that's how I felt on many days. My nights and, consequently, my periods of sleep, were shorter and less restful. I could see the changes in my appearance, and some days I felt so incredibly sad when I used to think of what we, as a happy, well-adjusted, and active couple, had been, and I wondered why it had all changed, why we were no longer that couple.

Despite the doctor saying that changes in Alzheimer's patients happen slowly over several years, I could see pretty rapid changes in my husband. The doctor was wrong.

My husband had little or no interest in anything; it was becoming increasingly difficult to carry on any semblance of a conversation. He was having difficulty even doing things, such as putting his socks on or going to the bathroom without some assistance. He often needed help in either finding the bathroom or in putting the toilet lid up.

I had to accompany him into the bathroom 90% of the time, either to assist him with clothing or to flush for him. When I didn't accompany him into the bathroom, I stood just outside the door with it opened a bit, so I could watch him for signs that he needed help. I often saw him smile and wave at the mirror, and his image reflected there.

One time, as he was looking into the mirror, he said, "I like that guy." I mentioned that to a professional, and she replied, "We don't know who he was seeing in there. It could be himself as a young boy, his father, or someone else that he liked and admired."

As a caregiver, you learn to multitask very quickly. You may have to interrupt cooking or eating to help your loved one to the bathroom, or to wipe up a puddle of urine when they didn't make it to the bathroom quickly enough. At first it seems difficult, but you soon become accustomed to it and then it's no longer troublesome and/or uncomfortable to pull on your rubber or plastic gloves to clean up a mess. You'll be surprised at what you are capable of doing, and doing it with good cheer when you are caring for someone you love and cherish.

There are times when you hold back tears as you are cleaning up broken pieces of a favorite vase that got knocked off the table during your loved one's nighttime wandering through the house. They don't even realize that anything has happened and, although you may be devastated to lose a favorite vase, you don't say anything to them. Why? Because you don't want to make them feel bad or that they've done something to displease you. So you hide the tears as you go on about your day.

No one can understand the degree of helplessness you feel when, in the middle of the night, your husband is walking the floor, wanting to see his mom and dad, both of whom have been dead for several years. There is nothing you can do when this happens or when he keeps saying, "I want to go home", and you can't make him understand that this is home... that he is home.

You soon learn that you can't convince, argue, or make someone with Alzheimer's understand, so you just agree with them or try to re-direct their thinking. This isn't always easy to do. And sometimes, you depend on the fact that they probably won't remember the conversation.

14

Going Through the Holidays

September begins the season of holidays. Many of us find ourselves celebrating Labor Day, Halloween, Thanksgiving and Christmas, as well as other special events and occasions. These last few months of the year can become quite stressful for the caregiver.

Despite feeling sad, lonely, and possibly even a little resentful, you accept the truth that the holiday seasons of previous years are no longer possible for you and the loved one you are caring for now. The years of family gatherings, dinners, outdoor outings, gifts, and laughter won't happen in the same way now. And, depending on how much you've done for preparations in the past, holidays or special events now will be different in how you prepare for them.

Of course, you will want to spend time shopping, cleaning, and cooking for every special day celebrated. But this extra work increases the possibility of you becoming more frustrated and of losing your patience. It also makes you tired and more apt to be a little short and maybe even cranky with others.

So, the question arises... how do I work all of this into my daily life as a caregiver? How do I incorporate all this into my already busy life? How do I take care of my loved one with all the distractions around me? How will all this extra activity affect them?

But your main concern is whether or not YOU can get through these days... are you strong enough physically and emotionally to get the extra work done and still take care of your loved one? You ask yourself, "Can I handle the additional stress created by the holidays?"

From my experience, I can tell you that this isn't going to be easy. But there are a couple of things you can do to help you get through it. Firstly, and most importantly, you MUST TAKE CARE OF YOURSELF!

Put simply, this means that you must get enough rest, eat a good balanced diet, and manage to spend some time outside the house and away from all the hubbub of the holidays. Go out for a walk, have a latte or a sandwich at your favorite coffee shop, read a book, write a letter, or just sit quietly and enjoy having some alone time.

Taking care of yourself also means accepting help from others. You may have to ask for support but do get it one way or another. If there are no family members nearby, then call on one of the agencies in your area that will be able to supply an aide for a few hours a day, several days a week. Friends and neighbors who genuinely care are usually willing and anxious to help however they can.

Be realistic about what you can manage. Consider simplifying your celebrations by cutting down on the number of guests, using an outside source for food, and possibly even hiring household help for cleaning, service, food, etc.

But above all... DON'T TRY TO DO EVERYTHING YOURSELF!

Give yourself credit for what you have accomplished and don't feel guilty if you lose patience or can't do everything on your own.

15

5 Caregiver Rules

One of the most vital things to remember when caring for someone is that they need to be kept safe and need to feel comfortable. Doing this is not always as simple as it sounds.

I learned several tips as I struggled with balancing the additional stress of holidays with my normal routine. Hopefully, these things will help you get through the holidays.

If you will have visitors to your home over the holiday, you need to make sure that your loved one is kept contented and, if they are physically able to, can participate in conversations or activities. Although you may enjoy having guests, remember that the person you are caring for comes first and that your time and attention must be directed mainly to them.

Although they don't mean to be a problem, visitors can change the dynamics and affect the atmosphere in your home. Your loved one may become agitated or even combative with the visitors when they speak loudly or touch them.

Consider your loved one and how they will feel being amidst a crowd. It is probably a good idea to limit the number of people around at any given time. Having visitors also puts an additional strain on you, and you may begin to feel agitated or otherwise distressed.

Be cognizant of the fact that your loved one may not know who the people around them are, and that the noise and/or activity may be frightening to him or her. Be sure to watch for signs that they are getting tired, nervous, or restless; they may just need to get away from it. In that case, you should simply remove them from the visitors or the situation.

If your loved one is incontinent, they may be embarrassed by 'an accident'. Be certain that you ensure visits to the restroom on a regular schedule or when you feel/sense they might need it.

If they have problems feeding themselves, make sure you make accommodations for them to have their meal in a private place. Also, make sure that whoever assists with feeding is someone your loved one knows and that your helper is aware of the established pace of eating and drinking. Do not rush this process or change it because of the holiday and the possibility of a very different menu that day.

If your loved one is in a facility and you decided to take them to your home for dinner or for opening presents at Christmas, remember that you need to keep a close watch on their reactions and be prepared to take them to a quiet room or even back to the facility if you feel it is warranted. Don't force them to remain in an environment where they are uncomfortable.

I have heard stories of home visits that were very difficult and often embarrassing for the person who was ill, for the family, and for others who were present. For example, your loved one might make inappropriate comments, have an outburst, or even have a urinary or bowel accident. They may spill food or drink, cry, or experience some other emotional breakdown. They may be disruptive and even aggressive. So be sure you know how your loved one will react in these situations before you decide to take them home for a special occasion. Consider it carefully before making a decision, a home visit may not be good for either of you.

Whether your loved one has Alzheimer's or another type of dementia, keep in mind that THEY CANNOT COME INTO YOUR WORLD, SO YOU MUST GO INTO THEIRS. This simply means keeping things comfortable for them and not expecting them to be able to socialize or even interact with others the same way they did when they were healthy.

Remember too that family and friends are often uncomfortable around someone who is ill. They may not know what to do or say. You also need to take their feelings and reactions into consideration when inviting guests.

It is a certainty that your frustrations and sadness will increase during special holidays/events, which is normal. Just try to keep in mind that you still have your loved one with you and that you can still enjoy the special times with them, albeit in a different way.

Each of us handles stress in our unique ways – you may choose to not participate in holiday celebrations, or you may limit your activities and keep as close to your regular schedule as possible.

Regardless of how much you choose to participate in holiday events, you will have several negative feelings during this time of the year. So when you feel alone, lonely, sad, concerned, irritated, hopeless, and maybe even a little resentful or angry, please give yourself some time to sit quietly and maybe even cry a little. Pray for strength and courage. Above all, don't show your frustrations to your loved one; just put on a happy face and go about your day.

Know that you are important in someone else's world, and also know that what you can do for them is to ensure their remaining days are comfortable, happy, and that they are kept safe. Although you will still have feelings that are sometimes hard to deal with, you can also feel proud that you are giving another person security and comfort.

So, just to refresh your memory, my Caregiver Rules 1-5 are listed below. Keeping them in mind can help you get through the holidays easier:

1. Always watch your tone of voice, keeping it friendly so that you don't appear bossy, critical, mean, or harsh.
2. Accept the challenge that has presented itself and then look for, and find, a workable solution.
3. Keep life as simple as possible while adjusting to the changes around you.
4. Look for, find, and savor, the good moments.
5. Live in the moment!

Rule #5 should be your guiding light not only during the holidays and other special times, but also every day as you go down the road that you and your loved one will travel during their illness.

16

Tinker, Tailor, Soldier, Spy...

My next blog post reads:

Tinker, Tailor, Soldier, Spy...

Tinker, Tailor, Soldier, Spy is actually the title of a best-selling book from a few years ago and none of these professions apply to me but that title keeps rolling around in my head, reminding me of the many hats I wear these days.

On any given day I wear the hats of housekeeper, cook, laundress, chauffeur, plumber, gardener, bookkeeper, financial advisor, dresser, barber, lawn care, planner, life coach, and on and on and on. How do I feel about all this? Frustrated at times, resentful at times, tired sometimes but always somewhat pleased that I was able to do all those things for someone I love, keeping his life together in the face of the Alzheimer's that has turned his world (and mine) upside down.

Since I have chosen not to write specifically about Alzheimer's disease and my husband's decline, but about my feelings as we travel down this path, I'd like to share some things now that would be difficult for me to sit down face to face with a friend to talk about. First, if I sat down to talk about it, I would probably stammer around and have trouble saying what I really wanted to say and secondly, I would probably cry. It's generally easier to write about strong feelings than to talk about them. So, here goes:

It's been a while since I last wrote anything on this blog, but I often thought about writing and really wanted to. However, I just didn't know how to explain my feelings/thoughts which changed rapidly as each day brought new challenges and were frequently jumbled and confused. I believe I have finally accepted what our life has become, and my feelings/thoughts have become clearer to me.

I have never had those "Why me?" thoughts and have never questioned that whatever we are experiencing is God's plan and that He will guide us through these trials. I have prayed, and continue to do so, that my words and actions will be what my husband needs at the time, that I am able to make him comfortable and that he knows he is loved and cared for. However, a few weeks ago I saw a friend and her husband in church and the feeling hit me that my husband and I would never be able to do those normal things again. Those friends are about the same age as us, why can't we have that kind of life? And I confess, at that moment in time, the "Why me?" thought crossed my mind.

Since that day, it has soaked in that we will not be able to do any of the things we used to do; we can't jump in the car for an impromptu golf weekend or even go out to the local course for nine holes on a pretty fall day; no getting together for dinner and cards with friends; no afternoons spent checking out a new shopping mall or outlet center; no more "date nights" with wine and a nice dinner and no more long discussions or conversations over dinner at our table. Nope, it's all gone.

Last night as we lay in bed, I put my arm around him and thought how I just wanted him back like he used to be. I wanted to see my generous, happy, strong, opinionated, loving, appreciative husband back. So how do I feel? Mostly sad right now.

My feelings have gotten stronger and more focused. As I said, I am feeling sad, often aggravated, and resentful, frustrated, and I also feel very lonely a lot of days and, sometimes I just feel all used up but then, thankfully, I rise up again and find something cheerful and fulfilling in my life.

There are good days when we laugh a lot, and he tells me how much he loves me. I try to show him my devotion through my care and by trying to keep things on a comfortable and calm level. We just had our 36th anniversary and special times like that are the times I miss my husband the most. I really, really miss the "us" that did so much together.

Say a prayer for both of us!

17

A Life that's Mourned

After that posting at the end of October, things seemed to worsen more quickly. He was now up almost every night till 2 or 3 AM, generally walking the floor, moving from room to room, sitting down on every chair and often moving chairs or other items around, sometimes even moving them to another room.

There were many nights when he became highly agitated, and insisted that he "wanted to go home." I would then take him out in the car at ten o'clock, eleven, or even midnight. Driving him around for thirty to forty-five minutes and then returning home, I'd hope that he would enter the house and feel like he had come home, and that he would then settle down for the night.

After doing this several times, I stopped because he sometimes wouldn't get out of the car when we came home. There have been many instances when after taking him out in the car late at night, I had to call his sister so she could help me get him into the house when we came home. While taking him out in the car at night might have seemed like a rather good strategy, it didn't work for long.

By then I had become such a light sleeper that I woke every time he got up, and mostly followed him around the house trying to convince him to come back to bed. On many occasions, I would make him toast and jelly, or a grilled cheese sandwich in the middle of the night. That usually soothed him and he would go back to bed and sleep. However, he would sleep till noon or later the next day, while I'd be getting up at 8:30 or 9:00 AM. I would start feeling exhausted pretty early in the day.

He would often lie in bed at night and talk about how we would go to Florida and play golf. He would also speak about his mom and dad, and about how he wanted them to come live with us. He would talk for quite a while, often patting me on the arm or leg as he spoke. Those were the times when I felt most helpless since I had to lie there talking and trying to show enthusiasm for plans that I knew were only dreams that could never come true.

I felt the loss of my husband and partner most acutely at those times – I would put my arms around him as I held back tears and silently prayed, "God, I just want him back!" But sometimes the tears would come anyway so I just hid my face, squeezed him tightly, and enjoyed holding him close to me. I don't think he ever knew how I was feeling – I didn't want him to know.

He experienced many of the symptoms associated with Alzheimer's; hallucinations, fear, incontinence, delusions, and sundowner syndrome. He slept a lot and, although I was concerned about the amount of sleep he was getting, I also appreciated having the quiet time for myself, time that I could spend doing things around the house or sometimes, just sitting down with a book or taking a nap.

By then, it had become difficult for me to even be in a different part of the house when he was awake. He liked me to be in the room with him and would frequently turn his head or raise up if he were lying on the couch to look for me. When I was out of the room, he would call out to me; he needed the assurance and safety of my presence.

We didn't go to the family Thanksgiving dinner that year. A niece brought dinner over to us.

This man who had previously been so outgoing and family-oriented was just not up to anything that took him out of the house and away from his comfort zone. It was a sad day, a turning point. I knew then that we would never be able to go back to any part of our old life of family celebrations and times spent together. I felt the loss keenly, and I spent the day quietly, almost as if in mourning.

In a way, I was.

18

Attrition

I was tired! Physically, mentally, and emotionally. I felt all consumed! I felt alone and helpless. I was also beginning to question my decision-making… was I doing the right things for him? Could I be doing something better? Could I somehow slow or stop the progression of this disease that has him in its grip?

I've realized that being a caregiver is no easy task!

I think it makes a difference when the one you are caring for is someone close to you. I'm no expert but I think that a caregiver can do more and with less hesitation when they know the person.

In fact, I found myself doing things that I didn't know I could do. Things such as cleaning up bathroom accidents; using a plunger (and sometimes even my gloved hands) to clear a blocked toilet, giving a bath which included washing private body parts, brushing teeth, giving enemas, inserting suppositories, etc. The list goes on and on. The need is there, and you somehow just find the strength and stamina to take care of it. You become conditioned to clean up messes without gagging or feeling nauseous.

But in between those duties that are sometimes distasteful and generally difficult to do, there are moments of smiles, laughter, hugs, and maybe even some meaningful conversation. These are glimpses of a former, pre-illness person. And, maybe, just for a little while you can even pretend that things are okay in your world. These moments are precious, so keep them close and bring them out to help you get through the bad times.

Sometimes during the day, I would look at him sleeping on the couch. I would look at his face, a face I have loved since the first day I saw him, and my heart would crack just a little bit more. Tears would slide silently down my face as I would whisper to myself, *'I just want him back, I want him back the way he used to be!'*

19

My Shrinking World

One day in 2017, while I stood at the kitchen sink doing dishes and looked out at the beauty of a summer day, I realized that I was not the same person I had been. That thought saddened me and added to the feelings of loneliness and despair that had, by then, become my constant partners.

I had always experienced happy feelings and joy when surrounded by the sunshine, flowers, and the smell of freshly cut grass. I felt happy when we sat in our gazebo late in the day, hearing the sweet birdsong that accompanied the otherwise quiet of the evening. But that day, standing there at the kitchen sink, I did not feel any happiness or joy. In fact, I felt no emotion except that of being tired, lost, and of not knowing who I was anymore.

My skin was dull – my hair dry and barely combed, and I wore no make-up, not even lipstick. I looked bad and not at all like myself. My life was consumed with caring for him and keeping things as close to normal as possible. I didn't have time for myself anymore.

I had always had a lot of interests; reading, golfing, writing, crafting, and working on my computer. I loved to take care of my garden, and I really liked to bake. I was a social person and had been involved with different groups in pursuing various interests. My husband and I had gone out a lot, enjoyed dinner, cards, or golfing with our friends. We also cherished each other and had some wonderful conversations.

But that day I felt the loss of the person I had been. Where was the care and pride I had always taken in my appearance? I missed having a soak in the bathtub or even getting a long hot shower.

My shrinking world now primarily consisted of being in our house. We had gotten to the point that most of our time was spent indoors, even on beautiful summer and fall days. I missed human contact and communication with others.

Visitors made him uncomfortable so I discouraged visits from everyone, except his sister and her family. He wanted me with him all the time and didn't like me talking on the phone for any length of time, so I also discouraged friends and family from calling.

That particular morning, as I stood looking out the window, I realized how small and secluded my world had become; I also knew that I had lost my contact with the outside world. I felt like we were isolated and out of touch. It was not a good feeling!

I felt the loss of my former self and I wondered… is this all there is? How do I find my joy and zest for life again? How can I be a good wife and caregiver when I can't even find myself? It was a frightening moment for me… how could I function normally when I didn't even know who I was anymore? I felt empty… all used up!

I realized later that I should have probably spoken with my doctor about my desperate feelings, but at the time that thought didn't even occur to me. I just kept it all inside and worried that I would lose myself, the person I had always been.

Even though it had taken me a pretty long time to realize that I was a caregiver, and quite a while to adjust to my shrinking world, it was a shock to now see how it was affecting me. My husband had always been my rock, my champion, my encourager, the one who made everything all right in our lives, and now he was no longer capable of doing those things. Since we had no children, I found that I was alone in making decisions and caring for him, our home, and our financial obligations. I wondered… where did caring for myself fit in?

All my original fears and doubts about my ability to take care of him and the tasks associated with our lives resurfaced. Now I also had a new worry… how could I find myself again? How could I find my way back into a normal world?

On any given day, I was likely to feel one or more of the following:

- Hurt
- Angry
- Frustrated
- Helpless
- Alone and/or lonely
- Incompetent
- Inadequate
- Lost
- Sad
- Hopeful
- Exhausted

I think the hurt, the sadness and the frustrations come with the territory, regardless of whether you are caring for your loved one at home or if they are in a care facility. Dealing with unexpected changes will absolutely cause these feelings, plus others that I haven't listed here.

The anger you will occasionally feel is toward the disease and the changes it has made in your life; it is not directed at the victim.

Seeing your loved one suffer the ravages of disease is hard and will, of course, affect your feelings. How we choose to deal with our feelings will often offer a path to conquering the changes to, and around, us.

Although it is normal for a caregiver to feel sad, frustrated, lost and lonely, it is also essential to keep reminding yourself that these feelings are normal and that it is okay for you to experience them. But also remember that you must find time to take care of yourself so you don't get lost in your shrinking world.

20

Questions that No Book can Answer

Things were getting worse. Around this time, he started repeatedly asking to see his parents. As I have previously noted, both of them had been dead for years. I told him it wasn't possible to see them since they both were gone. He asked where they had gone when I explained that they had died and were in the cemetery and he said, "Oh, you've bought into that crap." He still insisted that he wanted to get them and bring them to live with us.

This went on for weeks. Finally, one evening after he had already been in bed for a couple of hours, he got up and entered the room where I was sitting. He was wearing his coat and hat, and he insisted that we get his mother and dad. I said, "It's late, we can't go now." He stood there in the doorway and said that he would go by himself if I wouldn't take him. Not knowing how to handle this, I explained again that it was late at night but, thinking he would not remember, I told him we could go the next morning. That satisfied him, and he went back to bed.

Concerned with how he would be or if he would even remember my promise when he got up the following day, I got up at 8 AM and called the cemetery office. I explained to the woman who answered that my husband had Alzheimer's and was intent on coming over there to get his mom and dad. I told her I didn't know if I could talk him out of it and that if he insisted, I would have to bring him over as I couldn't take the chance of him trying to go there alone. She assured me that they would handle it gently if we came to their office. That relieved my mind. I could have hugged that nice lady!

Thankfully, he never mentioned it when he got up and, in fact, never mentioned it again.

But, once again, I realized there is no 'how-to' book that would lead me through these days. And I wondered, where could I turn when I needed answers? Who would help me realize what to do?

21

Strangers in Our House?

December came, and with it, a sharp decline in his condition. He was up every night, roaming around the house and sometimes being destructive without even knowing what he had done. The beautiful 1920's Victorian lamp that had belonged to my mother was knocked off the table one night and the top globe shattered. Seeing it lying on the floor, the bent and twisted base surrounded by pieces of the globe, was so disheartening. I quietly cleaned it up and never mentioned it. He would have been so upset had he realized what he had done.

Another night I found him sitting at the dining room table, pouring the oil from a liquid candle onto the table. Fortunately, I had the table pad on so there was no damage. It was like having an into-everything toddler around – I had to keep an eye on him all the time.

At this time, he was hallucinating regularly, thinking there were bad people in our house, people who wanted to kill us. He was very fearful, and I must confess, a few things he said made me wonder whether some of it was factual, like when he asked me where those people in our house had gone. When I mentioned that I didn't see them, he told me there were three of them, where they had been standing and even described what they looked like. I said they must have left because they aren't here now.

Later, when getting ready for bed, I went out onto our porch and leaned over the railing to make sure our garage doors were closed. Only to find that one of the doors was open and the overhead light was on. That unnerved me and made me ponder the possibility that someone had been in our house. After thinking about it for a while, I figured out that he had accidentally hit the light switch in the garage instead of the door closer when we came home from a quick trip to the post office earlier that afternoon. Even though that was a plausible explanation, the whole scenario was spooky!

He had a history of bowel impaction, and when symptoms appeared in early December, I tried Miralax, suppositories, and an enema to unblock him. He did not feel well and needed to go to the ER to get it treated, but he wouldn't agree to go. It was a long night and, for both of us, an exceedingly difficult one.

Around 2 AM, after I had pleaded with him all night to let me take him to the ER, he was in pain and walking the floor. Then he took off all his clothes and moved around the house, sitting on every chair and bed, leaving a brown stain wherever he sat. He didn't respond to my distress and just continued to sit naked in the living room.

By 4 AM, I just couldn't take it anymore and went into the kitchen where I beat my fists on the counter and simply stood there. I wailed. I <u>felt frustrated, overwhelmed, and completely helpless.</u>

I didn't know how I could stand the strong feelings of complete hopelessness and helplessness any longer; I felt utter despair that filled and consumed me at that moment and made me question my own sanity. There was absolutely no one that could help and nowhere to turn. That was the lowest moment of my caregiver experience. I wasn't sure I could survive it.

I settled down after a while and knew that calling 911 was my only choice, even though I knew he would never forgive me for that. They came quickly and were wonderful with him, although he was not cooperative and often was not even responsive to their requests. They finally got him into some underwear and a robe and, with lots of coaxing, insistence and help, were able to get him into the ambulance for the trip to the hospital. I rode with them in the ambulance and later called his sister to bring our car to the hospital so I would have transportation home.

Emergency Room personnel manually removed the bowel obstruction. It was a painful and scary procedure for him. I was by his side all the time, trying to calm and comfort him. It ended up being a horrible day as they sent him home while he was semi-conscious from the two injections they had given to relax him. Three of us – his sister, her husband, and me – couldn't get him out of the car in his unconscious state. I had to call 911 for the second time that day since we needed help getting him up after he fell to the ground as we tried to get him out of the car.

The paramedics came quickly, checked his vitals, and told me that he should not have been sent home from the hospital in that condition and that he needed to be taken back. After checking him and reviewing what they had previously given him, the ER physician administered another injection which was, as he explained to me, like Narcan. He said it would reverse the effects of the two drugs they had given him earlier to relax him. Scary!

Why am I telling you this? Because it had a lasting effect on him. Due to that painful experience, he became very protective of his rear end. He often wouldn't let anyone help him later on when he needed to be changed or cleaned up.

22

A Drastic Change Imminent

Aside from the terrible hospital experience, it was becoming very apparent that he needed more care than I could provide at home. And frankly, I was feeling physically, mentally, and emotionally exhausted. I was simply used up! There was nowhere to turn for help. I had no one!

Then, one night in mid-December, he refused to get out of the car when we returned home from one of our late-night rides. It was late, and no amount of my pleading convinced him to go into the house. Finally, at about 11:45 PM, I called his sister and asked her to come over to see if she could help. When she arrived, she managed to convince him to go in, but in the meantime, he had become very angry with me and refused to go in if I was there. So, my brother-in-law and I stayed outside, hiding behind the car so he wouldn't see us until he went inside.

Once inside, he sat down, still wearing his coat and hat. He refused to speak to anyone except his sister, but at one point, his anger suddenly switched from me to her, and he would no longer talk to her but only to me.

They left around 2 AM, but he continued to sit, still wearing his coat and hat and didn't speak the entire night. Around 7 AM, I was able to convince him to go to bed. When he awoke mid-afternoon, he didn't seem to remember anything about the problematic night we had. The incident was never mentioned.

After that night, I knew that things had gotten to the point that I could no longer take care of him at home, and to be honest, at that time, I was beginning to have some concerns for my safety. Since he frequently "saw" people in the house and would tell me that they were trying to kill us, I feared he might hurt me, thinking he was protecting me. I hid all the knives and sharp objects. His sudden anger at me that night was also a concern.

His sister and my son, as well as our primary care physician, recommended that I consider placing him in a facility. I wanted to keep him at home, and I resisted at first. But as things continued to slide downhill rapidly, I realized and accepted that the time had come when I couldn't take care of him and keep him safe anymore. I just didn't have anything left to give. I began looking for a facility the next day.

I was fortunate to quickly find a lovely Memory Care Assisted Living facility close to our home; I toured the facility, crying throughout my interview and subsequent tour of the facility. I made arrangements for him to move in.

Later that month, we had another incident. And at that moment, I felt relieved that I had made arrangements to move him to the care facility. I was already stretched well beyond where I was comfortable, and that night was just about more than I could handle.

23

I Have to Let You Go...

I was weighed down with guilt after I made the decision to place him in the facility. I dreaded the day when I would take him away from home... away from me. I could hardly bear to think about what that would mean to both of us.

I held him in my arms at night and told him how much I loved him; I recalled when we met and how, in that moment, I knew that I wanted to spend the rest of my life with him.

I was stunned when just before Christmas, they called to tell me that his move-in date would be December 27th. I thought I would have more time with him. It was now real, and the days were numbered for us to be together in our home. I felt guilty and questioned the decision I had made. I didn't know if I could do it... could I actually take him there and leave him? I changed my mind twice, but eventually, I accepted that a care facility was the best and only solution for both of us.

The day was drawing near – that dreaded day when I would take him to an assisted care facility. I could hardly bear to think about what that would mean for us. I realized that our life together would effectively be over. Nothing would ever be the same again...

While sitting at the breakfast table one morning the week before his move-in date, he commented that he 'felt like something bad was going to happen.' I don't know why he thought that and could only assume that he had heard me on the phone with the Long-Term Care Insurance Company or that he sensed my anxiety and concern since we were so close. Either way, I felt terrible for him, and I felt so guilty that I was about to take such a step, a step that would dramatically change his life and mine. However, I knew in my heart that I had no choice; things were just too unstable for me to continue home care.

24

A Cold Wind Blows

It was Christmas Eve, and it was 27 degrees outside; cold, snowy, and windy. I had to take him out in the car late that night. He was highly agitated and restless, and nothing I did seemed to calm him. We drove around for about 45 minutes. As we were driving down a quiet street, he accidentally opened the car door; that alarmed me, but I quickly pulled over, and we closed the door with no mishap.

Because of previous incidents, I had been apprehensive about taking him out that night. Although before we left our house, he had promised me he would get out of the car when we came home. When I pulled into our driveway as we returned, we sat there in the car for a few minutes before, with some coaxing, he finally got out and went into the garage. I was immensely relieved when he went inside.

The problem arose when he wouldn't leave the garage and go into the house. He stood there, looking out the windows in the garage door and standing between our two cars for about 45 minutes. I tried and tried to get him to come into the house, but he wouldn't budge. He wouldn't even talk to me, just stood there. I felt I had to stay in the garage with him since I feared he would go outside if I left him alone.

I didn't know what to do, I was cold even though it was about 45 degrees in the garage. Moreover, I was so exhausted. I had no other ideas about how to get him inside the house. Finally, in desperation and an act of helplessness, I leaned onto the trunk of my car, my head down on my arms, and just started crying.

After a while, he asked what I was doing, and I replied that I was crying and praying because I didn't know what else to do. Then, just a few minutes later, he quietly went into the house and proceeded to get ready for bed.

Even at his worst, he seemed to react to my tears.

As much as I dreaded taking him to the memory care facility, standing there in the chilly garage on Christmas Eve, I selfishly thought that December 27th couldn't come quickly enough for me. As much as I loved him, I realized I was totally worn out, and I couldn't go any further. I had to let him go.

25

You've Got A Friend In Me

Remember how you felt when you met that special person, the one you just knew was 'the one'? Remember the thrill of falling in love? Remember how you dreamed of having that person in your life always? Remember how dreams of building a home and family together filled your head day and night?

I remember those days vividly…

We were not youngsters when we met, and neither of us was the type of person whose head would fill with outrageous or unattainable dreams. Both of us had been married previously and knew what we wanted, and needed in our lives.

We both wanted a partner… someone to share our deepest thoughts and dreams with, someone who would understand our desires and be there for us in every situation. On top of that, we each desired to be loved, cared for, and treasured. We both had dreams of what we wanted a relationship to be.

After almost five years of dating, we started planning a wedding. We talked a lot and expressed our wishes for what we wanted our future to look like. Our wishes were simple, and we felt we could build the life we each wanted together.

Now, when our lives have been impacted so dramatically by his illness, I think back to those years of building our love and life together. Not a day goes by when I don't wish that I could have had more time with him. As it was, we had 38 years of marriage together, and those were good years! We never stopped dreaming, we created a wonderful life together, and when he became ill, I still dreamed of his return to good health and to spending more time together.

But in my heart, I somehow knew that our time together was limited by the Alzheimer's that robbed him of his world and, eventually, his life. The night before he went into the care facility, we laid in our bed, holding hands, as he talked about his wish to spend another winter in Florida. He said, "I think I could drive it; you can help me."

Knowing that there was no possible way we would ever travel again, I let the tears slide silently down my face as I talked with him to plan the trip I knew we would never make. That was one of the hardest things I ever had to do.

Oh, how I wished that we could turn back the clock!

But for that one night, he still had his dream and his wish for our future. He didn't know that things would never be the same for either of us again.

Our wishes and dreams of many years together are now treasured memories. Thank God for giving us the time together to build the beautiful memories that now sustain me.

26

The Two of Us

On moving day, he ate a good breakfast and was calm and sweet. I was sad and felt even more guilty about what I had to do. I had a difficult time keeping a smile on my face and forcing cheerful conversation. I hated to see the clock moving steadily toward the 1:00 PM appointment time.

I had previously told him that I had found a place where they might be able to help him 'find his words again', and he had agreed to go there with me for the appointment. Of course, he didn't know that he would be staying there.

When the time came to leave, he put on his coat and hat and walked through the entire house as if he were looking at it for the last time. He then walked downstairs toward the garage, but before he got there, he said he had to go to the bathroom and turned back into the house. After going to the bathroom, he sat down in a chair, still wearing his coat and hat and refused to move. I finally had to call his sister, who was able to talk him into getting up and into the car.

The staff was very welcoming and helpful. He was cordial and seemed interested as they showed him around the building. After a while, he said, "I'm tired; let's go home now." I told him I needed to go home to pick something up and that he should stay there; I would be back shortly. He was sitting on the side of the bed, and I encouraged him to rest while I was gone. His sister and I left him sitting there. We planned to come back at dinnertime to eat with him.

When we returned at 5:00 PM, he was in the hall outside his room, and he was livid! He was so angry at both his sister and me. My heart broke wide open as he looked at me and said, "How could you do this to me?" There was so much hurt and anger showing on his face as he said that. I tried to convince him that they would try to help him, but none of my words meant anything.

He just got more and more angry until his sister sternly told him that was enough, and he quieted down as he stalked down the hall away from us. I didn't know what to do… should I follow him and continue trying to settle him down? I started walking down the hall, just a little way behind him.

One of the facility's care partners was standing at the end of the hall. When I asked her what I should do, she said to just leave him alone, go home and that they'll take good care of him.

We left. It was heart-wrenching to walk out that door as we watched him walking down that hall, still wearing his coat and hat, so alone. I felt my heart shatter into a million pieces as we walked out.

My guilt resurfaced, and I wondered how I could have done that to him.

I have never been able to get that picture of him walking away, so alone and lost, out of my mind. I feel sick even today when I remember that night and the hurt and betrayal he must have felt.

Thankfully, his anger disappeared overnight, and he was in good spirits, interacting with other residents the following day.

Moving him into the Assisted Living facility was the single most difficult thing I've ever had to do. I knew he would never be home again, which was almost unbearable. Not only had I lost my partner and the love of my life, but I had also lost half of myself. While there was a certain relief in knowing that I was relieved of the worry and the work associated with his care, I missed him greatly.

When I pulled into our driveway that night, I began to crumble inside. I walked into the house where we had lived for 30 years, and it didn't feel like home without him. I felt like a stranger in my own house. I called my son and broke down, crying and talking with him and my daughter-in-law for over an hour.

I think I was in shock, and I started questioning whether or not I had made the right decision by putting my husband in a facility. Had I given up too soon? Was I being selfish? What would I do without him?

I spent another hour on the phone with my sister, crying uncontrollably.

I missed his presence; I missed seeing him. I missed everything. I felt so alone! I wondered what I would do without my other half, which was such an important part of me. My heart was broken… I never thought I would grow old alone. I thought there would always be the two of us.

Actually, I don't know what I'd thought – I just never imagined having to be without him. I thought we'd always be together.

27

The Things We Do for Love

Taking care of a loved one is hard! But you already know that by now.

Even though you know intellectually that there isn't going to be a good outcome for your loved one and that your struggles can't alter the situation, your heart still holds hope for the future. But there will come a day when you must face reality; when that happens, you will need to have your head and heart in alignment.

Alignment... what does that mean? It simply means that you will have to accept the harsh reality of the situation, both in your head (intellectually) and in your heart (emotionally). And believe me, you will be devastated when that moment comes.

So, how will that awareness affect you?

It will crush you! You have now realized that nothing you can do will have an influence on your and your loved ones' lives. It will most likely make you even more caring and attentive than before, but it won't increase the number of days your loved one is left with.

Although it is a painful thing to do, you must make sure to get things in order. You need to ensure that legal documents are updated so that wills and trusts accurately reflect the wishes of your loved one. Don't put this off for too long.

We had reviewed all our legal documents earlier in my husband's illness, and I felt comfortable with that decision at the end of it. However, it was only after I had moved him to the care facility that I conferred with our attorney about protecting assets. I should have done that earlier as it was, at that point, too late to transfer any assets out of his name. Regardless of whether you will be private pay or your loved one will receive Medicaid benefits, there are certain limitations as to whether, and at what point, you can transfer assets from your loved one to someone else.

You will want to make certain that steps are taken to protect your assets. In my situation, our attorney recommended that I make an appointment with an "Elder Law" attorney. I sat down with her to review my documents and discuss my concerns. She made recommendations to my attorney, and then the two attorneys worked together to review and, where necessary, to revise documents.

Seeing an attorney will, in all likelihood, cost you several hundred dollars, but unfortunately, it becomes a necessity.

I must also point out that if you are filing for Medicaid coverage, some different rules apply. You will need to determine the laws in Ohio, Kentucky, Indiana, or whatever state your loved one resides in. There are limitations regarding the amount of assets that can be retained by the person who will be covered by Medicaid. You should consult with an Elder Law attorney if possible and if not, contact the Department of Human Services in your area for information.

So, for now, and for all the days remaining with your loved one, just love them, kiss them, hold them, laugh with them, dance with them, read to them, and make them comfortable. Enjoy being with them. You never know how long you have with them.

Don't let them see your distress; do your crying privately, but let your feelings out. Talk to friends and let them help you through this stressful time. Pray for God's mercy and comfort for you and your loved one.

28

Was He Okay Out There?

I continued to have mixed feelings about whether I should have decided to place him in the care facility or not.

I realized that removing him from our home didn't dismiss my worry or my need to still be a caregiver. Oh, not at all! Now there was the additional concern for his well-being since I was not with him all the time. I didn't know what was happening with him.

Was he comfortable? Was he hungry? Was he safe? Was he happy? Lonely or frightened?

And I worried about whether his physical needs were being taken care of… was he changed when he had an accident? Did someone help him with the toilet? Were his clothes changed regularly? And I wondered, did he get his meds when he was supposed to? There was suddenly a whole new layer of worries for me.

One of the things the facility professionals told me was that now I could again be a wife and not a caregiver. Well, that did sound nice, but I knew in my heart that I would always be both a wife and a caregiver; I would always function in one role or the other as the situation warranted. I also realized that now I was his advocate and would function in that role consistently.

It was my duty to ensure that he was being treated with care and respect; that he was kept clean and well-fed; that his health was being monitored, and that he was being encouraged to participate in social activities that might possibly stimulate his brain and help push away the terrors associated with Alzheimer's or any other form of dementia.

I learned not only about the aides that worked in his area, but those in adjacent areas as well. I inquired about his eating and his sleeping schedules. I questioned whether or not he was taking his meds and whether or not he interacted with other residents and the staff that coordinated activities. The staff knew I was keeping an eye on every aspect of his life there.

Staying involved with all care levels is important, whether your loved one is at home or in a care facility. You will want to be there for the doctor's visits, physical and occupational therapy sessions, etc. You will also want to ensure that their nails are trimmed, haircuts are given regularly, and their dental needs are addressed. Most facilities have a podiatrist and a barber who visit patients regularly. Your insurance will most likely pay for medical care, but of course, you will be paying for other services.

He seemed pretty happy and well-adjusted. Other than Alzheimer's disease, he was in good health.

But while everything was going along smoothly for him, I was struggling. I was lonely and felt that I was caught on a merry-go-round. My days were all the same – mundane and monotonous. I did what I had to do and no more. But, on the bright side, I was looking better. I was getting more sleep, taking better care of myself, and once again, taking pride in how I looked. Visiting him daily and interacting with the facility's staff made me more aware of my appearance. I was always careful to have a smile on my face when I saw him.

But I had forgotten how to be alone, to be honest. I had never dreamed that I would grow old alone. Those feelings were still with me, but as time went on, I felt I was getting better every week. I still cried when I thought about the life we had and how it had changed. Some days I felt so sad for him; I just wanted to hold him in my arms and bring him back to the man I knew so well. I missed lying in bed with him, being able to snuggle when I felt cold.

I missed touching him...

There were days when the house felt so empty and cold without him, and missing him became almost unbearable. When I felt like this, I would go to his closet and hold one of his shirts close, hoping to smell his scent, the scent that was uniquely his, a mixture of his deodorant and soap, a fresh, outdoorsy smell. But, after a while, that fragrance was no longer detectable and losing him became more final.

Around that time, I had lunch with a friend who was also a psychologist. When he asked how I was doing, I told him about my feelings of loss, the guilt I felt, my anxieties, and I told him about the feeling of not being myself anymore.

He listened, asked a few questions, and then told me that I was experiencing grief, that I had begun the process of grieving the loss of someone I loved. I was stunned to hear this, but I knew in my heart that he had diagnosed my feelings correctly. I had always associated grief with the death of a loved one. But now I understood it is caused by loss, regardless of its reason.

29

Why Him?

By June, he had been in the facility for almost six months and was content there. I knew he was comfortable and that he felt safe. Yet I could see him sliding downhill, and I spent sleepless nights worrying about him and wondering if I could have done anything differently, if I could have done more, had I given up too soon?

He never once, during the sixteen months he resided there, asked to go home. In fact, he wouldn't even go out of the building when I tried to take him to a dental appointment a few months after he went there. Except for two different times when I was sick for two or three days each time, I visited him every day. He was happy to see me each day.

I missed him terribly; I cried often, and some days I felt so angry that he had left me with the responsibility of maintaining our house when I didn't know how to do some of the things that needed to be done.

Our nephew who lived about 4 hours away, called one night to check on me. I told him about feeling frustrated and angry at my inability to do some of the things that my husband had done so beautifully in the yard. He came down the following weekend and spent two days working in the yard. He showed me how to do some chores that I had not known how to do before and encouraged me to call him with any questions or concerns. He was a Godsend!

I was also worried about what would happen if my husband outlived our LTD insurance policy. If the monthly benefits ran out, how long could I sustain the costs of his care? Would I have to use up all our assets and end up penniless?

Above all, I wondered to myself, why had this disease struck *him*?

Then I would visit him the next day, and he would give me the sweetest smile, a hug, and a kiss; he would say that he loved me better than anything else in the world, and in that moment, all I wanted to do was cry. I hugged him back and assured him that I would always be there for him and that I loved him too.

The time we had together wasn't much, but it would have to do. I prayed that God would help us both as we climbed this mountain.

30

Limitations and Fears

The CAREGIVER RULES 1-5 that I've referred to are listed earlier in this book. Each of these rules came about after I found myself dealing with a tricky situation based on something I learned while struggling with that particular problem.

These rules will apply not only while caring for your loved one at home, but also after they are living in a care facility. More than one of these rules may apply to any given problem you face. Please use them or craft your own.

<u>Always keep in mind that those who suffer from dementia, Alzheimer's, or some other type, cannot come into your world any longer, so you must go into theirs.</u> This simply means keeping things comfortable for them and not expecting them to be able to socialize or interact with others in the same way they did when they were healthy.

Recognize their limitations and fears. Don't try to convince or force them to do something.

Here are a few helpful hints:

- Gently redirect if they lose their train of thought or wander off.
- Be patient and kind if they are struggling to communicate or to perform a task.
- If you don't understand what they are trying to say or do, show your interest by asking questions.
- Be gentle in both conversation and touch.
- Be patient and give them time to respond.
- Accept and validate their emotions instead of trying to change their feelings.
- Smile, stay calm and be positive.

31

The Big Band 40's

One of the things I learned early on was that my husband responded to my touch even when he was scared, unsettled or somewhat aggressive. After he went into the care facility, he often gave the care partners a hard time when they needed to change or clean him up. When I was there, I found that I could assist them by putting my face close to his and talking softly to him, whispering assurances and endearments while they took care of his needs.

Care Partners working at the facility told me my husband's heart rate and breathing slowed when he heard my voice. Just the sound of my voice alone helped to calm him.

You will undoubtedly find that your loved one responds positively to your touch and voice. Hugs, holding hands, and other casual touching are some of the ways you can show your love.

Experts say that social interaction with others and listening to music are two things that stay with dementia patients longer. You should use every opportunity to put one or both of these in play whenever possible.

My husband loved music, especially the big band, 40's music. I had always kept a radio playing in our house all day. After he went to the facility, I would often lie down with him, put his favorite Sirius XM channel on my phone and put my head on his shoulder or my arm around him. Sometimes we would talk, but more often, we just lay there, enjoying our time together. At those times, I would close my eyes and remember the many times we had lain in bed together, planning a vacation, discussing current events, or simply holding each other.

I also kept a small radio in his room at the facility and would turn it to a station that played soft, soothing music, and leave it on when I left. He liked that.

Those were the good times!

32

Savor the Good Moments

As the weeks and months passed while I was caring for my husband, both at home and later in the assisted living facility, I learned more about dementia and how it affected a person. I read books and sought information from our doctors and from the internet. Everything I learned was helpful to some degree. Still, most of my learning came from observing his actions day and night and from his reactions to things around him that were part of our daily life.

Caregiver's Rule #4 states, "Look for, find, and savor the good moments."

There will definitely be days when you can't find a good moment, but you have to keep looking and don't give up. Do the best you can with what you are given. Remember that your loved one is living a very different life from what they previously lived. They are now held captive by the disease. They probably feel confused, alone, and fearful, yet they most likely are not able to express those feelings to you. You must become adept at reading them, their actions, facial expressions, and whatever verbal clues they are able to give you.

Just keep in mind that there are still many good moments in your life, even though some days, finding a good moment may seem pretty far-fetched. Don't give up... keep searching for these treasures.

Maybe you'll find one in the middle of a tense situation – it could be a smile or a hug that comes unexpectedly. Perhaps it's a softness that comes into the eyes that appeared to be cold just a moment ago. When this happens, you've just found a treasure!

You'll also find unexpected treasures when your loved one smiles at you and tells you that you are nice. There's also a treasure to be found at bedtime when you tuck them in, and they look up at you, smiling as they gently touch your cheek.

But don't let me mislead you... you won't always find these moments. Sometimes you will feel rejected when your hand is pushed away or when a hug is not returned. When those disappointing and hurtful moments occur, just remember that the person you love is still there, in that broken body. Their love for you is intact even though they aren't able to express it to you with words.

Cry your tears in private. Talk about your feelings and hurt with a close friend or a professional. And keep in mind, you must stay strong and healthy and that you need to keep a solid footing as you go through each day. It's not easy, but it is necessary.

So, don't let those treasured moments slip past you... find and enjoy every one of them!

33

My Last Moments With Him

Towards the end of March 2019, when I went to visit my husband, I found him sitting in a wheelchair, his whole body jerking every few seconds. I had someone help me get him to bed in his room and I called for the director of nursing to see what was going on with him. She told me the jerking was caused by his brain misfiring and would probably settle down.

The jerking did stop later that afternoon, but he was never out of bed after that day. At first he talked, ate, and seemed pretty much himself, but for some reason, he was quieter than normal and slept more each day. He also seemed to be in pain, but no one could identify the reason for his pain even though the doctor saw him several times.

Some days he would just look at me with such softness and so much love in his eyes. He would often stare at me like he was committing my face to his memory. I would lie down beside him, turn the radio on to his favorite station, and hold him. I could tell he was completely relaxed and calm.

Other times I would pull a chair up close to his bed and talk to him. One day he looked at me for a long time and said, "I don't want to leave you, but I'm going to have to." For the next several days, he repeatedly told me that he loved me and kissed me back every time I kissed him. Although I didn't recognize it then, those days were the beginning of the end of our time together.

After about three weeks in bed, he would hardly eat, even though the kitchen would puree the food for him. He grew more and more quiet and slept most of the time. I learned then that people with Alzheimer's don't "forget" how to eat; their brains just can't tell them when or how to do it. By this time, he had lost a lot of weight and his once healthy, muscular body was now skinny with his cheeks sunken. He was, by then, going downhill rapidly, and there was absolutely nothing I could do to help him.

Hospice came in to evaluate whether or not he needed around-the-clock nursing. They began providing that care, bringing in a hospital bed for him. He had a hospice nurse with him all the time, in addition to the nurses at the facility. They were very attentive and helpful and charted everything. He began getting pain meds every few hours.

On Saturday, the 20th of April, the hospice nurse heard someone wish me a happy birthday and inquired if that was the actual day. I said yes. She said,

"Nothing will happen with him today. He wouldn't do that to you."

The following day was Easter Sunday, and I felt that with him having been raised a Christian, nothing would happen to him that day either. He made it through that weekend without any changes in his condition.

The following day he tried his best to say something to me even though he had not, at that time, spoken for at least a week. His voice was so low and so weak that I couldn't hear or understand him even though I put my ear close to his mouth. I felt that he was trying to tell me that he loved me and was saying goodbye.

On Tuesday, the 23rd of April, I felt compelled to go see him around ten that morning. When I arrived, one of the nurses stopped me in the hallway and said she was on her way to call me because they wanted my permission to put oxygen on him. I said yes. She hurriedly brought a tank to his bedside.

While she was doing all this, I went into his room and was shocked at his labored, noisy breathing. Although I didn't know it then, what I was hearing was a death rattle. It was frightening seeing him in such distress.

There were several people in his room; the hospice nurse and her supervisor, the care facility nurse, the hospice chaplain, and the social worker. Once the oxygen had been applied, his breathing settled down. I felt since there were so many people there, I was only in the way, so I left.

I knew it was a terrible time, and I felt as if the world had just stopped spinning. I didn't know what to do… where to turn.

My knitting group met on Tuesday mornings, so when I left him, I drove to the Coffee Shop where they would be meeting. I really needed to be with someone right then. I went in and found two of the knitters there. I told them what was happening and that I needed to be with someone at that moment. They cried with me and comforted me.

I knew things would never be the same again.

That afternoon at 2 PM, my regular visiting time, I returned to the care facility. He was resting quietly, his breathing quiet and pretty normal. I kissed him when I entered the room, and he puckered his lips. I said to the nurse, "He pursed his lips when I kissed him!" and she replied, "Oh, he wants to kiss you back. He's just too tired and too weak to do so."

I sat with him, rubbing his hands, his feet, his face, and talking to him all afternoon. His sister came and sat there with me. I walked away from the bedside so she could spend some personal time with him. She whispered to him, kissed him, and I think, said her goodbye. We left at 6:30 PM.

As I walked across the parking lot to my car, one of the nurses called out to me. She asked if I was coming back in, and I said, "No, I'm going home to eat something and get some rest". She replied, "Good. I don't think he wants you here right now. He's taking his final walk with Jesus, and soon, Jesus will send someone he loves to get him. I don't think he wants you to have that as your last memory of him."

Strangely enough, her words comforted me. I went home, had a light dinner, and sat watching some mindless program on the TV. Around 9:10 that evening, the phone rang. It was the hospice nurse saying that "he had transitioned." I asked, "Do you mean that he died?" She said yes, at 8:45 PM.

I immediately went to him. I was shocked when I saw the peaceful look on his face and noticed how it was so unlined and smooth; I was amazed at how calm he was. He looked totally at peace. The nurse said he had not been in any distress but had just taken a big breath and peacefully passed away. I felt relieved that he had an easy passing; God had answered my prayer asking for mercy.

The night he passed away, I stroked his face and kissed him for the last time. I felt the loss of his presence so intensely. He was such a big personality! He had a loud voice, a big laugh and a smile that made everything all right. Even in his illness, he had been my rock.

The funeral director came to get him. As he wheeled him out of the facility for the last time, the staff on duty that night lined the hallway to say goodbye, many with tears in their eyes. Others reached out to his sister and me with a pat on the shoulder or a hug. Their devotion to him was evident, and I knew they would also grieve his loss.

When I got into my car to go home, the realization hit me with a bang... my husband of almost 38 years was gone! What would I do without him? Despite my sadness at losing him, I also felt sad for myself. Sorrow was consuming me, and it felt threatening. Could I get through this?

The day I had long dreaded had come. How would I be able to bear not having him around? Could I function without his council, his support, and his love? Was I strong enough? Did I have the courage?

34

The Aftermath

Earlier I told you about the changes that occurred in our lives with my husband's illness, and how his illness either directly or indirectly affected us.

I'm sure that almost everyone will deal with personal and lifestyle changes during a particular time of their lives or, in some cases, all through it.

When changes do occur, we have to decide whether we will accept the change and adapt to it or we will reject it. Many will likely ignore it and everything involved with it. But sometimes, we have no choice in the matter; the decision of acceptance or rejection isn't up to us; it simply is what it is!

After adapting to the many changes I faced during my husband's illness, and in the years that followed his death, I now realize just how much these changes affected me. I can see how I've changed and grown from the old me into the person I am today.

The person I am today is different – not better than before or worse than before – just different.

I am a little quieter, a little more apt to feel blue; sometimes I choose to be alone instead of with others; I often feel sad; I am more prone to be late, and sometimes things just don't seem quite as important to me as they once were. Everything I see or hear reminds me of my husband in some way. But I know he is always with me.

Sometimes I feel cheated!

- Cheated that my husband was afflicted with a horrible disease that eventually took his life.
- Cheated that I don't have him here to tell me about his luncheon with friends or about his golf game.
- Cheated that I can't tell him about a book I'm reading.
- Cheated that I don't have him here to kiss me goodnight and to snuggle with me on a cold night.
- Cheated that I will have to grow old alone.

But on the other hand, I am thankful for so many things!

- Thankful for the 40-plus years of love and happiness that we had.
- Thankful for our families.
- Thankful for my many friends.

- Thankful for my curious mind that keeps me busy and gives me purpose. Thankful for my relationship with God.

But, let me get back to the changes that occurred in our lives over the past few years, which include:

- The illness that changed our lives so completely and gave me no choice but to learn and grow so I could provide care for my husband.
- The deterioration of our social activities.
- Weighing all the options and making the hard decision when it came time to place him in a care facility.
- Being alone in our house, which no longer felt like a home without him.
- Knowing the time was coming when I would need to prepare to sell our house.
- Taking care of legal and financial matters without the benefit of his input.
- Losing the comfort and security of the life we previously enjoyed.
- Being alone and having feelings of being inadequate for the challenges I faced.

When I tell you about the changes that occurred in our life and how those changes affected both of us, I must also tell you that we shared many happy moments during these stressful years.

One thing that never changed was the love between us, and that never wavered. His smile and warm hugs continued up until the last few days of his life when he was just too weak to hug me.

I kissed him goodbye when I left him the evening that was his last one on this earth. I whispered goodbye, touched his face, and told him that I loved him. I think he somehow knew that even death, the ultimate change, was not enough to destroy what we had together.

35

I Miss You...

Even though it's now been a while, I feel him close to me every day. I have a picture of us on my nightstand, and I often say good night to him as I turn out the lights and stretch out in bed, moving my foot over to touch him. Then I realize that he's not physically there with me.

I still feel like a caregiver! I treasure the time I spent with him during his illness. And even though there were many days and nights when I felt alone, all used up, helpless, and frustrated, I now smile thinking of the moments when we would lie in bed, and he would hold me while he talked about plans for our future.

I smile whenever I think about dancing in our kitchen and when I remember how, before his illness, he would sing along to the song 'I Love You' while holding my face between his hands. He loved the movie 'The Sand Pebbles' and never tired of hearing the theme song from that movie which was 'And We Were Lovers'. After his illness, he sometimes asked me to play the Matt Monro CD with that song on it when friends stopped by.

I miss being able to care for him. I often find myself looking up from something and expecting to see his face in front of me. I pray that I did everything I could to make his life happy and good, and that I did everything I could to take care of him as he declined.

Now I find myself paying more attention to birthdays, anniversaries, deaths, and other events, and I care about the feelings and the health of the person celebrating or mourning the event. I feel like a caregiver… I do care about others; I care about their successes and failures, their families, and their mental health when dealing with stress in their lives. I will forever offer my shoulder to cry on, my ears to listen, my time to console.

I will be a friend.

I pray that God will lead me to make a positive difference in the lives of those around me and, yes, I will continue to be a caregiver when it comes to matters of the heart.

36

Ode of the Broken Heart

How often in our lives do we feel our heart is breaking? You may have felt like your heart was breaking when your teenage boyfriend broke up with you, or maybe when your parents wouldn't let you go to that party that everyone else was attending. In addition, you can probably think of other times when you felt heartbroken but, in general, that feeling soon passed and whatever caused the feeling was forgotten. There was no lasting effect from that disappointment, and life continued on.

What exactly is a 'Broken Heart'?

Well, the definition is, "a state of extreme grief or sorrow, typically caused by the death of a loved one or the ending of a romantic relationship".

It is actually a condition with symptoms that may feel like a heart attack, with chest pain and shortness of breath. But in reality, it is caused by going through an emotionally stressful event and not by clogged arteries.

What to do when your heart is broken?

Although it's a terrible feeling that seems like it will never go away, once it sets in, it can crush you like a boulder. But have faith that it will get better with time. Be good to yourself, make new friends, get a new haircut, or buy some new clothes. Do something that makes you feel happy, even if it's only for a short time. Something I've found helpful is talking about my feelings or writing them in a journal.

I loved my husband for many years and, even though he's been gone for a while now, I still feel that love for him. I miss him with every fiber of my being. But that hasn't kept me from moving forward. I have many friends; I go to my knitting group, my writing group, and my art class. I play cards once a month and am generally busy with my crafts and my many interests.

My heart was broken when he was diagnosed with Alzheimer's. It cracked even more when I realized that I could no longer keep him at home, and it just opened wide apart the day I had to place him in a care facility. And on the day he took his last breath, and I realized that he was gone and that I would never again get to hear his big laugh and look at the face that I had loved so long and so well; my heart shattered completely. I was totally lost in the sadness and pain.

So, does a broken heart ever really heal?

I don't think so.

No, I don't think it ever heals completely. Whenever I hear a song that he liked, or see something that he would have enjoyed, I am overwhelmed with a renewed feeling of grief.

The pain and anxiety in my battered heart has never gone away; it just dulled after a while.

Have I moved forward? Yes, I think he would have wanted me to do that.

Does my heart ache? Yes, and I think it will ache forever, even though I am moving forward without him.

37

I Smile Because It Happened

When you were so bound up with being a caregiver, you probably never thought about stopping for a moment, just to be thankful. No, that was probably pretty far from your mind. You were so darn busy keeping it all together and so frequently overwhelmed by the feelings of frustration and loss that you found it hard to feel anything else.

I went through all those feelings, but sometimes, in the middle of a hectic and frustrating day, when I was feeling hopeless and pretty much helpless, I realized that I had so much to be thankful for.

Yes, I said thankful!

Even though my life had changed dramatically with my husband's illness, I realized that I could be grateful that he was still there with me. I could see him, talk to him, touch him, kiss him, hug him, and help him when he was unable to do things for himself.

And I was thankful for my health and resilience.

I was thankful for the home we had lived in and loved for over 30 years, and I was thankful for the love and laughter we had shared. I felt gratitude for the family gatherings we had enjoyed, the holidays, birthdays, and other special days we celebrated.

In the years that I was taking care of him at home before moving him into the care facility and during the sixteen months he spent in that facility before his passing, holidays and special occasions were literally just another day for us. I felt sad and missed having family time, but when he became ill, my priority was taking care of him and making his life as normal as I possibly could. He just didn't remember the significance of any holiday or special occasion so, to him, those days were just the same as the ones before or after them.

Since he passed away, I now spend my holidays alone, but I've made it through each year even though I've often depended on visits to the cemetery and lots of tears to get me through the day. I've had bad days and nights when I wished it were possible to turn back the clock to our happy days. But I know this can't happen, so I try different things to assuage my feelings of sadness.

Sometimes I write letters to him, letters that recount our happy days. Some days, like yesterday, when missing him consumed me, I went to the closet, pulled out his favorite jacket and held it to my face. Although I can no longer smell his scent on the jacket, it still provides me some comfort.

Sometimes at night, I pull his pillow close, and I can almost feel his warmth. Often, I remember a particular moment and enjoy it again; I will whisper good night to his face smiling at me from the picture on the table next to my bed, and sometimes I dream.

A few months ago, on one awful night when I was feeling alone and lonely with no purpose in my life, I prayed to God to help me. I woke up the following day with the Serenity Prayer on my mind; I was repeating it over and over to myself, and I thought that was strange until I realized it was the answer to my prayer.

God was reminding me that we can change some things in the end, but we do need to accept the things we can't. WOW! What an awakening! I couldn't change the fact that my husband had died; I couldn't change the fact that I was alone. But I needed to accept that he wasn't coming back, and I also needed to accept the responsibility for my future happiness and contentment.

That realization didn't take away my sense of loss, my missing him, or my sadness, but it did help me understand that I still can enjoy life and look forward to special occasions and holidays again. I believe I have learned an important lesson from the Serenity Prayer... a lesson that I always need to evaluate things in my life, change the things I can, and accept those that I can't change. I also have to keep reminding myself of this prayer.

The Serenity Prayer was written in 1932-33 by Reinhold Niebuhr and is often quoted. It has been adopted and popularized by Alcoholics Anonymous and other twelve-step groups. I have printed it here, hoping that you will benefit from reading it.

God, grant me the serenity to accept the things I cannot change,
Courage to change the things I can,
And wisdom to know the difference.

Nothing can take away the years of worry and sadness that I, and many others, have experienced as we were caregivers for someone we loved. But when that period of our life is over, we need to learn to move forward into a new phase of our lives. It's not easy, but it is necessary.

With that being said, I hope you, like me, can make changes that will enable you to move forward with life, even though sometimes that seems impossible. Believe me... you can exist and live a good and happy life as you begin to evaluate and make changes or find acceptance.

Although my experiences as a caregiver for my husband were often difficult and painful, and even though at times I still feel guilty and wonder if I did everything I could, I am thankful that I was there for him when he needed me the most.

I believe I made his journey through illness easier just by being there for him as his caregiver, and I believe he knew how much I loved and treasured him, right up to the end of his life.

Whether you are caring for someone with Alzheimer's or any other type of disease or illness, or for someone who, although not impaired mentally or physically, is suffering through changes that may be part of the normal aging process, I hope you have found something in reading about my experience as a caregiver that will be helpful to you.

Keep in mind that medical science, as advanced as it is, cannot duplicate a hug, a kiss, or your presence. Also, remember that through displays of your love, attention, and devotion, you represent safety and security to the person who is suffering from illness and confusion.

Whether you are beginning, continuing, or ending your role as a caregiver, always remember that <u>you are strong, courageous, and capable</u>. Even though some days may be challenging to get through, you <u>will</u> figure out how to get through them.

Yes, <u>you</u> are absolutely capable of performing everyday miracles in your role as a caregiver.

Pictures of Al and Me

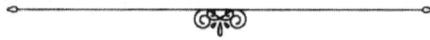

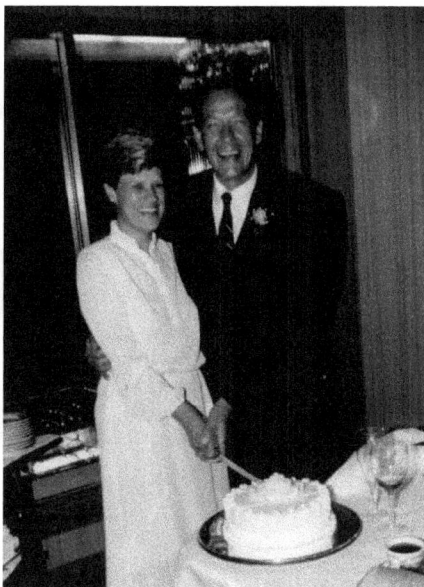

Our wedding on September 24, 1981

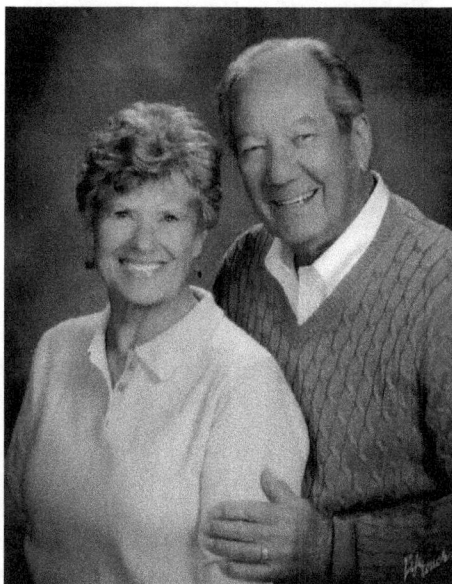

The first time we started noticing some memory issues in November 2013

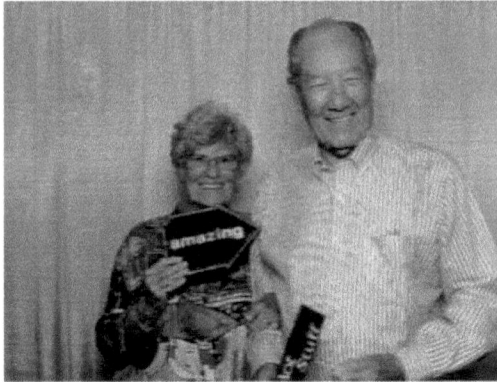

This picture was taken just a couple of months before his diagnosis in June 2016 – you can see how he has changed in appearance since the 2013 photo

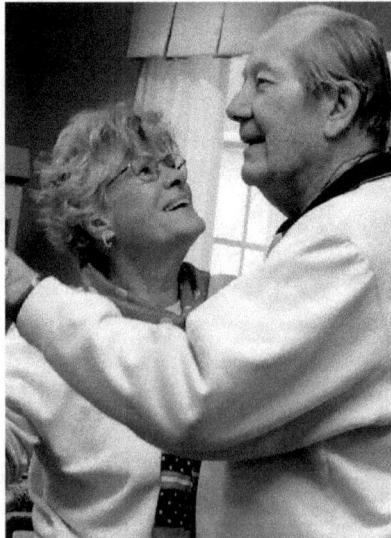

Valentine's Day 2018 – about 6 weeks after Al went into the Memory Care Facility where he was for 16 months

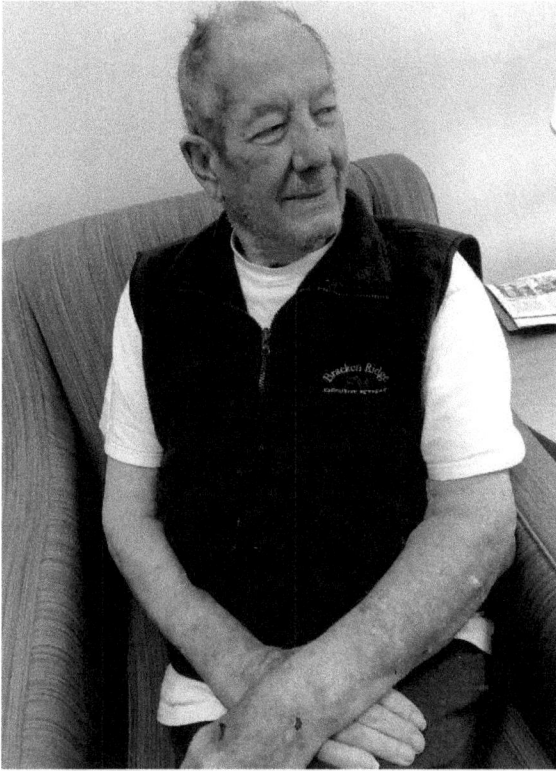

Al, circa end of 2018 or early 2019, about 3-4 months before he passed away on April 23, 2019.

About the Author

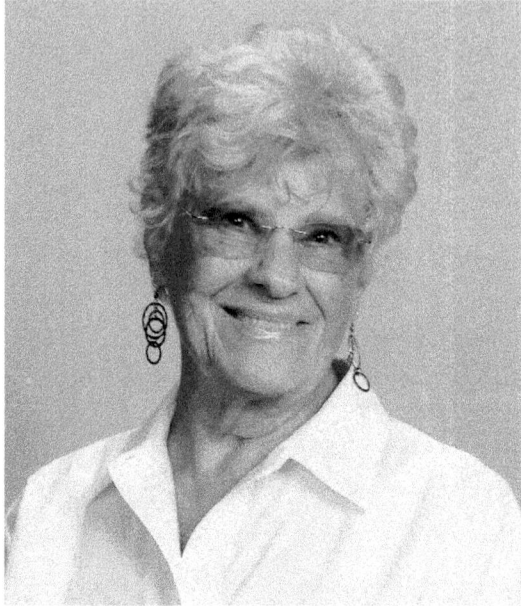

Jenny Zimmer, as the primary caregiver, provided care for her husband for several years. Through her role as caregiver, she learned a lot not only about the disease but also about how to handle the raw feelings, the stress, and the loneliness that comes with the process of watching someone you love decline. She hopes that through sharing her experiences, she can help others who find themselves in the role of caregiver.

Jenny is a retired Human Resources executive who now spends her time writing, painting, enjoying cards, mahjong, and dominoes with friends. She also volunteers at a local Assisted Living Memory Care Facility. Jenny's story, poem and essay collection 'A Carpet of Violets and Clover' & her poetry publication 'All the Moments are Real' are available on Amazon and Barnes & Noble in ebook and print.

Note from the Author

If you like what you read in this book, you can check me out on Facebook: (www.facebook.com/authorjennyzimmer) or Instagram: (@jennyzimmer5). If you have any questions, comments or feedback, you can also send me an email at jennyzimmer519@yahoo.com.

Review the Book

If you have time to post a review, that would be highly appreciated. You can do it on Amazon or any other online bookstore you purchased this copy from.